The Art and Science of Beauty Therapy

A Complete Guide for Beauty Specialists

Edited by Jane Foulston, Fae Major, Marguerite Wynne

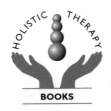

HOLISTIC THERAPY

BOOKS

Published by Holistic Therapy Books
An imprint of Ruben Publishing Ltd.
8 Station Court, Station Road, Great Shelford,
Cambridge, CB22 5NE
Tel: 0870 242 7867
Fax: 01223 846445
© Ruben Publishing Ltd 2007.

First published July 2007

Reprinted October 2007

ISBN 978-1-903348-08-6

Set in 10/12 Swiss Light

Printed by Scotprint, Haddington

Prepared for the publishers by The Write Idea, Cambridge

Acknowledgements

Our thanks go to Steiner Leisure and Elemis, in particular to Robert Schaverien Manager Director and Penny Hallworth Training Manager for the use of their superb training facilities and all the arrangements on the day of the photo-shoot. Additionally we would like to thank the Steiner students for their time and professionalism, and for taking time out from their hectic training schedule to pose for the photographs required for our book.

We would also like to thank the following for their assistance in providing illustrations for this book:

Angela Barbagelata, The Carlton Group

Caroline Morley, The Wellcome Trust

Amanda Robinson, illustrator

Contents

The editors

Jane Foulston

Jane Foulston has been in the beauty therapy industry for over 26 years. Jane taught beauty and complementary therapies in both further education and the private sector for 14 years. She also set up a beauty therapy college in Japan. Jane worked nationally and internationally as an ITEC examiner and took over as the Director of ITEC in 1998. Since then ITEC has gone on to become the largest international awarding body for beauty therapy in the world.

Fae Major

Fae Major has worked in the beauty therapy industry for 23 years. Her experience has included working for Steiner's, alternative medicine clinics as well as private beauty salons in the UK and Barbados. Fae has 15 years' teaching experience and as a result became a practical examiner for ITEC in 1992. As well as continuing to examine, Fae is currently working for ITEC as part of the Qualifications Development team.

Marguerite Wynne

Marguerite Wynne began her career in one of London's foremost beauty salons and went on to teach in the College of Beauty Therapy in the West End. Subsequently she owned her own salon and school in Buckinghamshire and at the same time worked as Chief Examiner for ITEC. In 2005 Marguerite was appointed Education Manager for ITEC where she now monitors the standards and consistency of ITEC examinations.

Introduction

A successful, competent and responsible beauty therapist must work to stringent professional, aesthetic and scientific standards. This book will help you to understand the key role of professionalism in your practice, to master the art of beauty therapy and to understand the scientific principles on which your therapies are based.

All these skills are not just about you, the beauty therapist, and your knowledge of your profession – they are designed to place your clients' welfare, safety and well-being at the centre of your practice.

Chapter 1:
Being professional

In this chapter we'll be looking at the following key topics which, together, combine to create professionalism:

Topic 1:
Professional appearance

Topic 2:
Providing a professional environment

Topic 3:
Professional communication

Topic 4:
Professional client care

Topic 5:
Professional health and safety

Topic 6:
Safety, risk assessment and the salon

Topic 7:
Professional record keeping

introduction

As a therapist you represent both your profession and your employer and, when clients consult you, they are placing their confidence in you as a professional. They are entrusting their health and wellbeing to your care, and they expect every aspect of the service you provide to be professional.

Being professional is about making sure that everything – including your personal presentation, communication and behaviour; the environment in which you work; client care; health and safety and, of course, the treatments you provide – all meet the highest professional standards.

Topic 1: Professional appearance

Within the first 15 seconds of meeting, your client will make a number of judgements about you and your abilities, all of which will be based on your attitude and your appearance. For example, if you look untidy and dishevelled a new client may make the assumption that the service you will provide to them is going to be slapdash and careless. However, if you look neat and well groomed, a new client is much more likely to assume that your treatments will be careful, competent and professional.

> KEY POINT
> Your appearance should confirm to your clients that you are a professional and qualified therapist and should give them the confidence to enable them to relax, knowing that they are safe in your hands.

Personal presentation

To ensure that you look professional throughout your working day you need to pay careful attention to the following:

1. Personal hygiene
Personal hygiene is a key element of professional presentation. Use a deodorant or anti-perspirant to prevent body odour. Always check that your breath is fresh and sweet smelling on a regular basis. Also ensure that your hair is clean and tied back off the collar and face and that your nails are short, clean and without nail polish.

2. Uniform
A clean and freshly ironed uniform is essential to presenting a professional appearance. If you are working in a salon you will be expected to wear professional work wear. If wearing white at work you will almost certainly need at least three uniforms; one to wear, one to wash and one to keep at work as a spare just in case you have an accident. Nothing looks more untidy or unprofessional than a white uniform that is marked with splashes or stains. It's worth noting that, for reasons of hygiene, many employers will expect you to wear tights or stockings, even during the hot summer months. If you wear tights, do make sure that they are plain and a natural colour.

If you are working as a sports therapist, the usual uniform is a polo shirt and tracksuit bottoms. If you are wearing trousers you should choose full, flat shoes and socks of the same colour. It is important always to make sure that you look neat and well groomed.

3. Hair
Hair must be clean and tied back from your face so that it doesn't flop forward or rest on your collar. Tied back hair will be cooler and more comfortable for you, and will also be more hygienic for the client.

4. Nails and hands
Nails and hands must be kept scrupulously clean. Nails should be neatly trimmed and unvarnished, unless you are a nail technician, in which case your own nails should be regarded as a valuable advertisement for your skills, and maintained accordingly.

5. Make-up
Make-up must be worn and should always look fresh and professionally applied.

6. Perfume

Heavy perfume should be avoided as some clients may find strong odours unpleasant, or may even be allergic to certain fragrances.

7. Shoes

Shoes should be practical and, above all, comfortable as you will be wearing them throughout the working day. Your shoes should have closed toes and heels, and must be flat. As you are likely to be on your feet for long hours it's a good idea to ensure that you have a suitable spare pair that you can change into halfway through the day. This will help to keep your feet fresh and comfortable. It's also a good idea to have spare socks or tights to hand so that you can change those as well if you need to.

8. Jewellery

Jewellery must be kept to a plain wedding band and small stud earrings. Dangling earrings, bangles and rings must be avoided at all times as they are unhygienic and may even injure your clients. Wrist watches should be removed and left in a safe place until the end of the day, but fob watches may be worn on your uniform.

Did you know?

Jewellery must be removed or covered if you are using electrical equipment.

KEY POINT

Never, ever, chew gum or suck sweets whilst talking to, or working with, a client. This applies throughout the premises and, if you want to maintain the best impression with your clients, outside the premises as well.

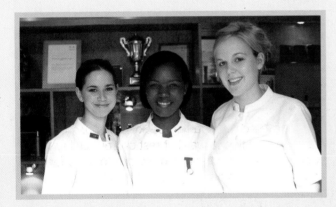

CHECKLIST

This checklist provides a set of quick professional appearance checks that you can run through at the start of the day and before each client.

Before you meet your client check that:

- ☐ your personal hygiene is beyond question
- ☐ your uniform is spotless
- ☐ your hair is clean and neatly tied back from your face and collar
- ☐ your hands are freshly washed, and your nails are clean, neatly filed and unvarnished
- ☐ you are wearing appropriate make-up, and that it looks fresh and professionally applied
- ☐ you are not wearing heavy perfume
- ☐ your shoes are comfortable, your socks are clean and your tights are not holed or laddered
- ☐ your jewellery is, at most, a plain wedding band and/or a pair of stud earrings.

A word about punctuality

Your client is entitled to expect that when they arrive for their appointment their therapist will be ready and available to begin the treatment. If you are late and keep your client waiting this sends a clear message that you do not consider them to be your number one priority. Many clients, quite rightly, will feel upset and irritated if their treatment doesn't start on time.

Also, your employer will expect you to complete a treatment within a commercially acceptable time. For example, in most salons, it is considered to be commercially acceptable to provide a facial massage lasting for one hour, and the price set for that treatment will be based on the cost of one hour of the therapist's time, plus the cost of salon overheads such as lighting, heating, products used, and so on. If, though, the therapist spends longer than an hour providing a facial massage this will have an effect on the business – if fewer clients than expected are treated during the course of a day this means less money going into the till. This, in turn, will affect the employer's profits, and their ability to keep the business running successfully. In addition, clients often have busy schedules and plan carefully to fit a beauty treatment into an hour. If the therapist draws out the treatment so that it takes longer than an hour, this can have a knock-on effect on the client's plans for the rest of the day, and make them late for other appointments. What should have been a soothing and relaxing experience can, if it takes too long, turn into a frustrating and irritating event which spoils the remainder of the client's day. This is not good for the reputation of either the individual therapist, or the business.

Keeping to time is an important part of professionalism. If you find that you are regularly running late with clients – which means keeping the next client waiting – you need to reflect on why this is happening, so that you can address the problem. Some points that can help you keep to time are to make sure that you do not:

☐ draw appointments out by chatting too much

☐ forget to keep an eye on the clock

☐ overestimate how much you can do in a given time.

Always remember that, after one client leaves, you will need a few minutes in which to prepare the treatment room – and yourself – for the next client.

END POINTS

By the end of this topic, you should understand that:

☐ being professional is about earning and keeping the trust of your clients

☐ your appearance should confirm to your clients that you are a professional therapist whose personal hygiene and presentation is beyond question

☐ you should know the time allocated for each treatment, and stick to it

☐ if, for any reason, you have to keep a client waiting make sure that you apologise sincerely, and assure them that the delay was unavoidable and will not happen again

☐ if you find that you are running late on appointments, think about why it happens, and address the issue so that the delay is not repeated.

Topic 2: Providing a professional environment

As well as making sure that your own appearance is immaculate, it's vital to ensure that your treatment room, and everything in it, is spotlessly clean, neat, tidy and ready for the client's treatment. Needless to say, no client wants to find themselves in a treatment room which looks untidy or unhygienic. And, from the client's point of view, nothing appears less professional than settling down for a treatment only to find that the therapist has to leave the room to gather extra supplies or to find a piece of equipment that is in safe working order.

CHECKLIST

As one client leaves and before the next client arrives check that:

☐ the treatment room is spotlessly clean, neat and tidy

☐ you have opened windows to allow in fresh air, or used an air freshener, if necessary

☐ any bins are emptied before the next treatment

☐ your equipment trolley is clean

☐ you have sufficient supplies of all the products you need for the next treatment – e.g. fresh towels, tissues, cotton wool, products, etc.

☐ any equipment you intend to use is clean (and sterilised where necessary) and in perfect working order

☐ you have your client's records to hand or, for a new client, you have a new record card ready to be completed

☐ you have checked around the room to make sure that, in your professional opinion, everything is in order and ready for the next client.

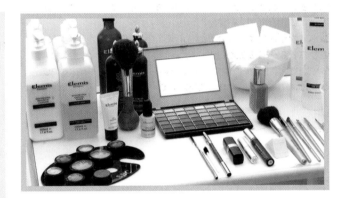

The client will judge the quality of the service you provide on their complete experience with you. Even if the treatment you provide is perfectly satisfactory, if a client judges that some other aspect of the environment is unacceptable – for example, unhygienic or untidy – then they'll probably look around for another salon that provides a cleaner, more pleasant, more comfortable setting for their next treatment. In other words, you are quite likely to lose a client to another business.

Salon hygiene

Providing a hygienic environment is a duty we have to our clients. It is also, for your clients, an important criteria by which they will judge your services, and whether or not to return or to recommend you to their friends and acquaintances. Good salon hygiene is a continuous process that will, if carried out properly, ensure that all areas of the salon, and all equipment used within it, are clean and free from contamination.

Preventing infection means ensuring that micro-organisms (organisms that are so small they cannot be seen with the naked eye) such as bacteria, viruses and fungi do not have the opportunity to survive and multiply.

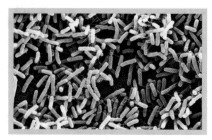

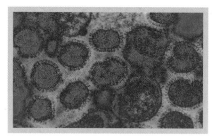

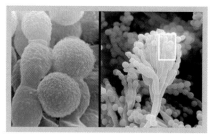

Bacteria

Bacteria are tiny have a range of shapes – round, rod-like, or flagellate – and only about one thousandth of a millimetre across.

While bacteria can play a beneficial role in parts of the ecosystem, may even provide antibiotics, and can help with our digestion, they are a cause of diseases ranging in severity from upset stomachs to pneumonia, tuberculosis and typhoid fever.

Viruses

Viruses are about a tenth the size of bacteria – indeed there is even one group, called bacteriophages, that feeds upon bacteria. They are responsible for some of the most devastating diseases of plants and animals. In humans, they are responsible for ailments from the common cold to herpes and HIV.

Fungi

While fungi can be seen (and enjoyed) as mushrooms, they are generally microscopic, and are another infectious organism that may affect us and our clients. They are responsible for the rising of our bread and the production of penicillin, but they are also the causes of ringworm, thrush, athlete's foot and fungal nail infections.

Type of infection	Characteristics	How it spreads	Examples
Bacterial infection	Caused by bacteria, which are single-celled micro-organisms	Bacteria reproduce at the site of the infection – skin, ear, throat, vagina etc.	Skin infections such as impetigo (staphylococcus pyogens) or acne (propionibacterium acnes) Food poisoning such as salmonella
Viral infection	Caused by viruses, which are micro-organisms smaller than bacteria. Viral infections do not respond to treatment with antibiotics – penicillin etc.	Viruses reproduce inside human cells	Common cold Cold sore – herpes simplex Chicken pox – herpes zoster Wart – verrucae Hepatitis A and B HIV, which can lead to AIDS – Acquired Immune Deficiency Syndrome
Fungal infection	Caused by parasitic growth, which includes moulds, rusts, yeasts and mushrooms	Fungus is reproduced by spores	Ringworm – tinea pedis, capitis or corporus Thrush – candida albicans

Did you know?
Unchecked, some germs spread so fast that they can double in number every half hour... so just one germ might become half a million in the space of a working day – hence the importance of regular and frequent attention to effective hygiene procedures in the salon.

Preventing infection and contamination

A client can pick up an infection from equipment that has not been properly cleaned and sterilised, or from products that have deteriorated with age or have been contaminated by another client.

To prevent the spread of bacteria, viruses or fungus within your working environment it's vital that you take the utmost care to ensure thorough sterilisation and sanitisation. This will ensure that no cross-infection occurs between one client and another. A variety of sterilisation methods and techniques are available for use in the salon. Here are some of the most suitable.

Autoclave
An autoclave is an item of electrical equipment which is used to sterilise small metal items such as eyebrow tweezers and scissors. When water is heated at normal atmospheric pressure, it boils at 100 degrees centigrade. The autoclave heats water under pressure, which increases the temperature at which the water

boils. At a pressure of 15 pounds per square inch (psi) the boiling point of water is raised to over 120 degrees centigrade – a temperature at which good sterilisation can be achieved in 20 minutes. An autoclave, especially one with an automatic timer and a pressure gauge, is simple and effective to use and economical to run. Items to be sterilised must be capable of withstanding the heat in the autoclave, and this method is suitable for metal instruments. It is vital that all items are washed or wiped prior to being placed in the

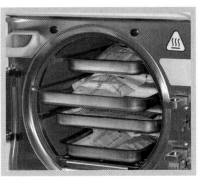

autoclave to ensure that all surfaces are free to be cleansed.

Disinfectant liquids and solutions
We are all familiar with the use of disinfectant liquids and solutions in the home, and appropriate products have a valuable role to play in the hygiene and safety of our salons. In salon use, a disinfectant must be effective, economical to use and inoffensive. Typical salon products are either chemical disinfectants that may require dilution according to their instructions for use, or alcohol-based disinfectants that may be used in the form of liquids, wipes, or gel-based hand washes. Examples include products such as Barbicide or Milton.

Before using any disinfectant product remember to:

☐ select an appropriate product for the use to which you are putting it

☐ clean before disinfecting

☐ follow the instructions

☐ wear appropriate safety equipment

☐ allow enough time for the product to work.

After use, remember that used products will be contaminated and no longer effective, and so should be disposed of carefully. Also bear in mind that some products, such as alcohol or gel hand cleansers may be flammable.

Ultraviolet radiation (UV)

Short wave ultraviolet radiation can be used to sanitise small items such as brushes and electrodes. The article to be sanitised is placed in a cabinet but must have already been cleansed. The UV radiation kills micro-organisms on the surface of the article. The UV radiation is only effective on the surface of items being sanitised (as it cannot pass through them) and, as light travels in straight lines, items must be turned during the process so that all surfaces are exposed to the light. The process takes roughly twenty minutes, and has the added benefit of not heating the item.

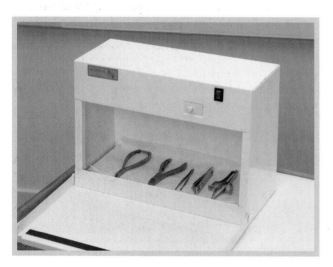

Chemical sterilisers

Liquid chemical sterilisers are plastic cabinets, usually with a perforated tray on their base. Most salon materials can be sterilised by cleaning and drying them thoroughly and then immersing them in the liquid chemical in the steriliser. After the time indicated on the manufacturer's instructions has elapsed (usually 10 – 30 minutes), the items can be removed and should be thoroughly rinsed. It is very important to choose the correct chemical for your sterilisation needs. The chemical requires changing after the time specified by the manufacturer, usually about 14 to 28 days. Be very careful to avoid skin contact with the chemical.

Hot bead steriliser

Hot bead sterilisers are small and easy to use. They are suitable for sterilising small objects but not for brushes, plastic, sponge or glass. Tiny glass beads are contained in a protective insulated case and heated to 190–300°C (375–570°F) as indicated by the manufacturer. Sterilisation takes between 1 and 10 minutes.

Did you know?

Until about 100 years ago, half of the deaths in developed countries were the result of infections.

How infections spread

Infections are spread by touch, food, water droplets in the air, and through contact with cuts and grazes and other kinds of skin abrasions. Although it is almost impossible to create a completely sterile environment, you can reduce the risk of spreading infection by:

- ☐ not treating clients who have an obvious infection or, if the area infected is small, by avoiding it
- ☐ sterilising equipment
- ☐ disposing of waste safely
- ☐ maintaining the highest standards of hygiene.

CHECKLIST

Ways to ensure a professional level of salon hygiene

- ☐ All hard surfaces – floors, worktops, trolleys, toilets, washbasins etc – should be daily washed down with a disinfectant /sanitiser
- ☐ Clean bed linen should be used for each client, or the treatment couch should be covered with clean couch roll for each new client
- ☐ Clean towels must be provided for each client, and towels should be laundered daily

- ☐ Clean towelling robes (if used) should be provided for each client

- ☐ Towels, blankets, towelling robes etc. should be laundered daily and then stored in a closed cupboard or laundry bin

- ☐ Waste bins should be emptied after each client and at the end of each day and disinfected

- ☐ Broken glass or used needles should be disposed of in a sharps container as the contents are collected and professionally incinerated

- ☐ If a client has any open wounds or abrasions on their skin you should avoid touching these areas, and should make sure that the wounds are covered with a plaster before the treatment starts. The same applies to the therapist.

Cross infection between clients can be prevented by:

- ☐ using disposable spatulas for waxing, etc

- ☐ placing a small amount of product – blusher, foundation, cleanser, etc. – onto a clean palette/ spatula for each client; never using fingers to decant products

- ☐ not scraping back into the main container any product that has been in contact with either your hands or any part of the client

- ☐ Used cotton wool, tissues etc. should be immediately disposed of in a covered waste bin

- ☐ Washing your hands thoroughly before and after every treatment is a must.

Thorough hand washing means:

- ☐ using an antibacterial soap or bactericidal gel and warm, running water

- ☐ washing forearms, wrists, palms, backs of hands, fingers, between fingers and under fingernails

- ☐ rubbing hands together for at least 10–15 seconds

- ☐ using a clean towel or a disposable paper towel.

CHECKLIST

Health and hygiene terms you should know

- ☐ **Antiseptic:** a chemical used to reduce the growth of bacteria

- ☐ **Asepsis:** clean and free from bacteria

- ☐ **Disinfectant:** chemical used to destroy bacteria not their spores

- ☐ **Non-pathogenic bacteria:** bacteria which are harmless or even beneficial to the human system, for example: lactobacillus acidophilus which is found in yogurt, and lactobacillus casei which is found in many cheeses

- ☐ **Pathogenic bacteria:** bacteria which are harmful and which cause diseases such as cholera, typhoid and tuberculosis

- ☐ **Sanitise:** make clean

- ☐ **Sepsis:** severe illness caused by overwhelming infection of the bloodstream by toxin-producing bacteria, which can originate anywhere in the body

- ☐ **Sterilise:** make clean and completely free from bacteria and their spores

END POINTS

By the end of this topic, you should understand that:

- ☐ infections caused by bacteria, viruses and fungi can easily spread from one client to another

- ☐ a client can pick up an infection from equipment that has not been properly cleaned and sterilised, or from products that have been contaminated by an infected client

- ☐ good salon hygiene is a continuous process

- ☐ thorough hand washing is essential to good hygiene as it will prevent the spread of any infection, and keep you and your clients safe.

Topic 3: Professional communication

As a beauty therapist good communication skills are at the heart of your ability to relate to your clients and to deal with them professionally. By using good communication skills you will encourage your client to relax in your care.

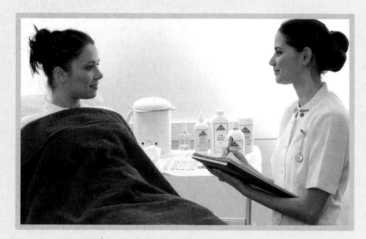

These skills include:

- ☐ asking the right kinds of questions
- ☐ listening with attention and interest
- ☐ being comfortable with silence
- ☐ using appropriate body language.

This, in turn, will contribute to their enjoyment of the treatment and should encourage them to return.

Asking the right kinds of questions

Asking questions is one of the best ways of encouraging clients to communicate with you – giving you the information you need to treat them effectively.

When asking questions it's important to understand the difference between **closed** and **open** questions, so that you can ask the right kind of question at the appropriate time.

Closed questions are those to which your client will be able to give a short Yes or No answer. Examples of closed questions include:

'Shall I open the window to let some air in?'
'Are you warm enough?'

'Would you like another blanket?'
'Have you had a facial massage before?'

Open questions can't be answered with a Yes or No. Open questions invite your client to provide information and to answer in detail. Examples of open questions include:

'What do you hope the treatment will achieve for you?'
'Tell me about how you sleep?'
'Which parts of your back are most stiff and sore?'
'Tell me about your diet?'
'How have you been feeling since the last treatment?'

KEY POINT

Open questions are particularly useful when:

☐ you are meeting a client for the first time and need to take their history and complete their client record card (see Topic 7: Professional Record Keeping)

☐ you are talking to a client you have seen before and you want to find out how they responded to the last treatment you gave them and if there have been any changes, problems or improvements.

Listening with attention and interest

Listening to your clients with genuine interest and attention will put them at ease and will help to build a good professional relationship between you. On the other hand, not listening to your client may persuade them that:

1. You are not interested in them

2. You don't care whether or not the treatment you provide is appropriate for their needs

3. You do not have a professional attitude to the work you do.

Listening with attention and interest involves:

☐ being focused on your client throughout the time they are with you and concentrating on what they are saying

☐ listening without interrupting

☐ making eye contact with your client whilst they are speaking

☐ asking open questions to find out more

☐ remembering things your client has said to you so that at the next appointment you ask them about what they have told you – their holiday plans, family wedding, changes at work, new pet and so on.

Did you know?
When a client hesitates before answering a question it is usually because they are trying to decide whether or not to tell you something important. Remember to give them time and encouragement … and to listen very carefully.

Being comfortable with silence

Some clients will enjoy talking throughout their treatment. They will regard the communication between you and them as an important part of the process, and they will happily chatter away about family and work and holidays and, probably, every other topic under the sun. Other clients, though, will regard their treatment time as a little oasis of peace and silence where they can simply relax and enjoy their therapy without having to make the effort to talk.

Once you have obtained any information necessary from the client, e.g. 'How have you been?'; 'Are you warm enough?' 'Would you like another cushion under your knees?' If the client lapses into silence, don't feel that you need to make small-talk. This may be the only time during a busy working week when your client has the opportunity to completely relax and allow them-selves to drift in peace and quiet. Don't spoil it for them.

Using appropriate body language

It is really important that you use appropriate body language with your clients, as this will put them at ease and reassure them that they are in the hands of a professional therapist.

Did you know?
Non-verbal communication is another name for body language.

Appropriate body language includes:

☐ smiling

☐ making eye contact

☐ sitting facing your client during conversation

☐ leaning forward slightly when talking to your client.

You also need to be able to read the body language of your client. For example, frowning, grimacing or raised eyebrows usually indicate that someone is irritated, uncomfortable or ill at ease.

Did you know?
The words you say are only a small part (7%) of the communication that takes place between you and another person. 38% of your message is communicated in how you say it, and a striking 55% is communicated through your body language.

END POINTS

By the end of this topic, you should understand that:

☐ the elements of good communication are being able to:
 – ask the right kinds of questions
 – listen with attention and interest
 – be comfortable with silence
 – use appropriate body language
 – make yourself clearly understood.

☐ open questions are used to gather information, whereas closed questions are used to elicit a simple 'Yes' or 'No' answer

☐ listening with attention and interest will put your client at ease and make them feel valued and respected

☐ using positive and encouraging body language will help your client to relax and enjoy their treatment

☐ paying careful attention to your client's body language will help you to see when, even if they don't say anything, they are feeling uncomfortable or ill at ease.

Topic 4:
Professional client care

Your clients have the right to expect a professional standard of care whenever they receive a treatment from you. Providing a professional standard of care involves:

☐ recognising contraindications

☐ taking account of your client's need for modesty and privacy

☐ not making false claims

☐ only providing those therapies in which you are fully trained and qualified

☐ not offering a diagnosis of any kind.

SALON NAME
Client Consultation Form – Make-up

Client Name: Date:
Address:

                                                      Profession:
e-mail: Tel. No: Day
                                                               Eve

PERSONAL DETAILS
Age group: Under 20☐ 20–30☐ 30–40☐ 40–50☐ 50–60☐ 60+☐
Lifestyle: Active ☐ Sedentary☐
Last visit to the doctor:
GP Address:
No. of children (if applicable):   **Date of last period (if applicable):**

CONTRAINDICATIONS REQUIRING MEDICAL PERMISSION – in circumstances where medical permission cannot be obtained clients must give their informed consent in writing prior to treatment. *(select if/where appropriate):*

Medical oedema☐	Skin cancer☐
Nervous/Psychotic conditions☐	Slipped disc☐
Epilepsy☐	Undiagnosed pain☐
Recent operations affecting the area☐	Whiplash☐
Diabetes☐	When taking prescribed medication☐
Other:	

CONTRAINDICTIONS THAT RESTRICT TREATMENT *(select if/where appropriate):*

Fever ☐	Scar tissue (2 years for major operation and 6 months for a small scar) ☐
Contagious or infectious diseases ☐	
Diarrhoea and vomiting ☐	Sunburn ☐
Under the influence of recreational drugs or alcohol ☐	Hormonal implants ☐
	Recent fractures (minimum 3 months) ☐
Skin allergies ☐	Sinusitis ☐
Eczema ☐	Neuralgia ☐
Trapped/Pinched nerve affecting the treatment area ☐	Migraine/Headache ☐
	Hypersensitive skin ☐
Inflamed nerve ☐	Botox/dermal fillers (1 week following treatment)☐
Undiagnosed lumps and bumps ☐	Conjunctivitis ☐
Localised swelling ☐	Stye ☐
Inflammation ☐	Eye infection ☐
Cuts ☐	Watery eyes ☐
Bruises ☐	Hyper-keratosis ☐
Abrasions ☐	Any known allergies ☐

SKIN TEST *(select if/where appropriate):*

Moisture content:	Excellent☐ Good☐ Fair☐ Poor☐
Muscle tone:	Excellent☐ Good☐ Fair☐ Poor☐
Elasticity:	Excellent☐ Good☐ Fair☐ Poor☐
Sensitivity:	High☐ Medium☐ Low☐
Skins healing ability:	Excellent☐ Good☐ Fair☐ Poor☐
Skin tone:	Fair☐ Medium☐ Dark☐ Olive☐
Circulation:	Good☐ Normal☐ Poor☐
Pores:	Fine☐ Dilated☐ Comodones☐ Milia☐

Recognising contraindications

A contraindication is a sign, signal or symptom that tells you that it would be unsafe to provide a particular kind of treatment or part of a treatment for a client:

☐ It might be unsafe for the client and could perhaps aggravate an existing illness.

☐ It might be unsafe for you and for everyone else in the salon.

Quite often the client will freely disclose, before the treatment starts, that they have a medical problem such as very high blood pressure or a heart condition. Many clients with all kinds of medical conditions benefit greatly from massage and other therapies that you are able to offer. But do make sure, in order to protect your client's health and safety, and your own reputation and the reputation of your employer, that you obtain approval prior to providing treatments.

Sometimes the client will not even be aware that there is a problem and it will only be when they have settled themselves onto the treatment couch that you notice something like recent scar tissue, severe bruising or what looks like a contagious skin infection.

Where there is a skin infection which could be contagious it's vital that you do not continue with the treatment as you could be at risk of:

☐ catching the infection

☐ spreading the infection throughout the salon.

However, it may only be necessary to avoid the area of infection not the whole person. Where you notice recent scar tissue, varicose veins, small cuts or abrasions, for example, it is fairly easy to work around these areas, making sure not to use any oils or other products or apply any pressure to the affected areas.

Contraindications can be classified into two different types:

1. Medical – your client has a medical condition, e.g. high blood pressure or diabetes.

In these circumstances you need to obtain medical permission from the client's doctor before you can proceed safely with the treatment.

2. Contraindications that may restrict the treatment

Beauty therapists should be able to understand and recognise those contraindications relating to beauty treatments requiring medical approval.

Where the client is unable to obtain such approval from a medical practitioner, the therapist needs to get 'informed consent' in writing from the client, which means that the client is made fully aware of the situation prior to giving any treatment for those contraindications that restrict treatment.

Contraindications for specific beauty treatments can be found in the following chapters of the book.

Taking account of your client's need for modesty and privacy

It is safe to say that, with few exceptions, most people (both men and women) have issues about one or more parts of their body.

For example, many women would like to have larger or smaller breasts, smaller waists, flatter tummies, thicker hair, smoother skin or daintier feet. In the same way, many men would like to be taller, more muscular or slimmer around the waist. The key point here is that, for some clients, the notion of removing their clothes and allowing a stranger to work on unclothed areas of their body may be quite daunting. It is therefore extremely important that you take account of your client's feelings throughout the treatment, and in particular ensure that your client's modesty is preserved at all times.

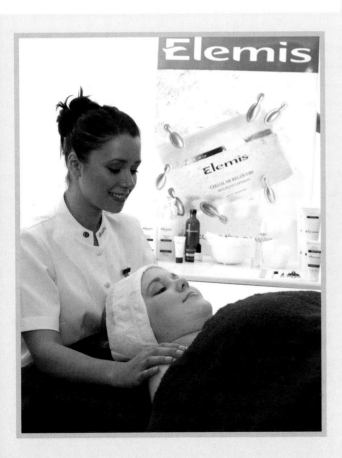

CHECKLIST

To ensure that your client's modesty is protected at all times:

☐ before the treatment starts explain to a new client firstly which areas of the body you will be working on and secondly the garments they will need to remove. Also reassure them that they will be completely covered throughout the treatment apart from the small, specific area of the body that you will be working on at any one time

☐ allow your client to undress alone and in complete privacy, and make sure they have a clean, unworn robe to wear as they walk to the treatment couch

☐ once the client is settled on the treatment couch wrap them in a blanket and towels. This will preserve their modesty, keep them warm and also provide a feeling of being cosy, safe and completely covered up

☐ when carrying out an intimate treatment such as an underarm or bikini wax, always provide a modesty towel and if, for example, you want the client to position protective tissues, always allow them to do this for themselves

☐ ensure that the client's privacy is protected at all times by making sure that no-one else can see into the treatment room. If, for some reason, another therapist enters the room during the treatment ensure that your client is fully covered so that their modesty is preserved whilst the other person is in the room. Even if the visitor is another therapist they are not your client's therapist and the client may feel embarrassed or uneasy.)

☐ make sure that your client has time and privacy to get dressed before your next client arrives

Remember, your client is entitled to be treated with the utmost respect at all times – before, during and after their treatment.

Not making false claims

As a professional you are required to work within the law. The Trades Descriptions Act 1968 relates to the false description of goods and making misleading statements to members of the public. What this means for you, as a therapist, is that:

☐ If a manufacturer makes a misleading statement with regard to their product – for example, 'Will make you look 10 years younger' or 'Will burn away all unsightly fat overnight' and you repeat the misleading statement to a client, you will be liable to prosecution

☐ If you make false claims about pricing – e.g. 'This moisturiser is a great deal because we're offering it at £10 (half price) this week' when it actually cost £15 last week you could be liable to prosecution.

Imagine, for example, a client asks for a particular treatment and says 'I've heard this is really good and smoothes out all lines and wrinkles.' If this is not true you will only remain within the law if you, for example, either agree that it is a popular treatment, agree that you've heard some clients have had good results, or agree that the product smells nice, or is very pleasant to use (providing that all these statements are true), and that the client could certainly try it for themselves and see what they think of the results.

It is fine to say what you are aiming to achieve with your treatment or therapy, and what you hope might happen as a result. But it is really important not to make promises about the outcome the client should expect.

If you make unrealistic or untrue claims you are breaking the law and, almost certainly, your client will be disappointed and unhappy when your false promises fail to materialise.

To stay within the law you must NOT:

☐ supply information that is in any way untrue or misleading

☐ falsely describe or make false statements about products or services

☐ make false contrasts between previous prices and current prices

☐ claim that a product or service is being sold at 'half price' unless it has been offered at full price for at least 28 days prior to the 'half price' sale.

Did you know?

The Advertising Standards Authority states that adverts should be legal, decent, honest and truthful. This means that salon owners and their therapists should not make any false claims about any of the products, services or treatments provided to clients.

It's also important to be careful and diplomatic when discussing other therapists and other businesses. It's quite likely that, from time to time, a client will ask you for your opinion about another therapist, another salon, or even a therapy with which you are not familiar. Always make sure you say nothing that is discourteous or detrimental to another person or business. Making false or damaging comments is both unprofessional and dangerous as you could find yourself in court facing a case of libel.

Only providing those therapies in which you are fully trained and qualified working within your own scope of practice

As a professional it is vital that you recognise your role and its limits. From time to time a client may ask for, or you may feel tempted to offer, advice or treatment in an area in which you are not trained or qualified.

Don't go beyond your own limits. Always stick to what you know, and remember that you are in a relationship of trust with your client. If you go beyond the limits of what you can or should do, you are breaking that trust and may also be risking harm to your client. Always remember that if a client in your care is harmed then your own career and reputation may be damaged, possibly beyond repair.

In a situation where a client asks you for a treatment which you are not able to provide don't hesitate to refer them to a more experienced therapist. In these circumstances, always make sure that you have the client's permission before passing on any details of their treatment and health.

Not offering a diagnosis of any kind

In your career as a beauty therapist there will almost certainly be times when a client will ask 'Will you have a look at this … what do you think it is?' The client might be asking about a lump or a mole, a lesion, a patch of dry skin, a rash …. there are any number of different possibilities.

No matter what you think or suspect, it's vital to remember that you are not trained or qualified to diagnose. Regardless of the circumstances do not offer your opinion but do suggest that the client consults their own doctor. You can do this without alarming the client by saying something like 'To be honest, I really don't know what it is. If I were you I'd make an appointment to see your doctor or your practice nurse … they'll be able to have a look and tell you what it is.'.

END POINTS
By the end of this topic, you should understand that:

- a contraindication is a sign, signal or symptom that tells you it would be unsafe to provide a particular type or part of a treatment to a client.

- a contra-action is a sign or symptom that a client has responded unfavourably to a treatment or a product.

- when necessary, you should not hesitate to refer clients to their GP, practice nurse or another professional if you suspect they have a medical condition which needs attention.

- you should never offer a client a diagnosis, even if they ask. You are not trained or qualified to do this.

- you must always recommend only those treatments which are relevant and appropriate for the client.

- you must never offer treatments or advice outside the areas in which you are trained and qualified (scope of practice).

- you must never make false claims for the treatments you provide, or the products you use.

- you must avoid making disrespectful or damaging comments about other therapies, therapists or salons.

Topic 5: Professional health and safety

No matter where you work, under the law, both you and your employer have a number of health and safety responsibilities.

Did you know?

Your employer, regardless of the size or type of organisation where you work, has a legal responsibility to provide:

- a safe and healthy workplace which is kept in good condition
- equipment that is safe to use, e.g. scissors, computers, stepladders, tanning beds
- safe systems and procedures of work
- at least one person who is competent and trained to supervise health and safety at work.

You have a legal responsibility to:

- co-operate with your employer's health and safety requirements, procedures and policies
- follow safe systems of work – e.g. using equipment safely and following instructions for the use of products
- not interfere with or misuse any equipment or protective clothing provided by your employer
- take care of your own health and safety, and the health and safety of your work colleagues and your clients.

Health and safety legislation

The main law on health and safety at work is:

- ☐ the Health and Safety at Work Act 1974 (sometimes referred to as HASWA).

The most important regulations which cover health and safety at work are:

- ☐ the Management of Health and Safety at Work Regulations 1992
- ☐ the Workplace (Health, Safety and Welfare) Regulations 1992
- ☐ the Provision and Use of Work Equipment Regulations 1992.

Basic first aid

Every business is required, by law, – the Health and Safety (First Aid Regulations) 1981 – to ensure that there is First Aid provision available to deal with accidents and emergencies at work.

In large companies there may be very sophisticated first aid facilities with trained personnel and a dedicated first aid room. In most small businesses, though, it is considered sufficient to have:

- ☐ one person on the staff who is the appointed person who can take charge in an emergency situation – e.g. calling for the fire brigade, or an ambulance. The appointed person should receive Health and Safety Executive approved emergency first aid training, and also refresher first aid training every three years

- ☐ a first aid box which is kept well stocked with appropriate items

- ☐ an accident book in which all incidents can be carefully recorded.

Emergency situations involving work colleagues or clients can happen at any time. For example, someone at work might faint, burn or scald themselves, twist their ankle, have a nose bleed or start to bleed profusely from a cut, be stung by an insect, become dizzy, have an asthma attack or an epileptic fit, start to hyperventilate, fall into a diabetic coma, receive an electric shock or have an allergic reaction to a product you are using on them.

Even though you may not be the appointed person for dealing with accidents and first aid emergencies, it is vital that you understand what to do if an emergency situation occurs.

Did you know?

A risk assessment is the process of:

regularly carrying out a careful examination of the workplace, equipment and work systems and procedures to identify hazards and potential hazards

identifying and removing, or making safe, the hazards and then deciding whether or not any further action needs to be taken to eliminate similar hazards in the future

taking further action as appropriate – maybe reorganising workspaces, arranging additional training for staff, changing working practices, etc.

A hazard is something that could cause harm to someone. Examples of hazards include:

electrical plugs that have not been properly wired

treatment couches that are in need of repair or replacement.

sharp scissors that are left lying around, and inappropriate disposal of sharp objects.

A risk is the chance that a hazard will cause harm to someone, for example:

electrical plugs that have not been properly wired so that when you plug in the electrical appliance you receive a shock and, possibly, severe burns

treatment couches that are in need of repair or replacement so that when a client lies down the couch gives way and collapses. The result being a very shocked client who may even sustain injuries such as a sprain or broken bone

sharp scissors that are left lying around so that when a work colleague accidentally bumps into the couch where the scissors have been left, the scissors fly off and embed themselves in her arm.

CHECKLIST

Dealing with a first aid emergency

If someone at work, either a colleague or a client, becomes ill and appears to need medical help:

- ☐ immediately find the person who is the appointed person/first aider, and follow their instructions.

- ☐ if the person who has been taken ill cannot, in your opinion, be safely left on their own, get someone else to find the appointed person.

- ☐ if the appointed person is not in the building, dial 999 (112 within the EC). You can make this free call from any telephone, including your own mobile.

- ☐ Ask for the ambulance service and provide the information that the control officer on the other end of the line will ask for:

  - – your telephone number and your location
  - – the type and seriousness of the incident: e.g. someone has fainted, or scalded themselves very badly
  - – details of the person involved in the incident: sex, age, condition, etc.

- ☐ If necessary, the control officer will pass messages on to the other emergency services such as the fire brigade and police.

The recovery position

If someone is unconscious, there is a safe position which you can put them into which allows them to breathe easily and stops them choking on any vomit. This is called the recovery position.

In an emergency situation, if the appointed person isn't available, you may have to put a client or colleague into the recovery position. To do this:

☐ check their airway is clear

☐ check they are breathing

☐ check they have a pulse

WARNING!
The casualty may have head or neck injuries. It is therefore very important that:

☐ you ensure the person's head and neck are supported at all times

☐ you do not allow rotation between the head and spine

☐ you do not tilt the head back if you suspect there may be a neck injury.

CHECKLIST
How to put an adult into the recovery position

1 Position casualty's legs:
☐ kneel beside casualty

☐ straighten casualty's limbs

☐ lift nearer leg at knee so it is fully bent upwards

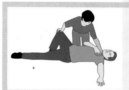

2 Position casualty's arms:
☐ place casualty's nearer arm across chest

☐ place farther arm at right angles to body.

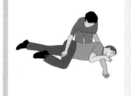

3 Roll casualty into position:
☐ roll casualty away from you onto side

☐ keep leg at right angles, with knee touching ground to prevent casualty rolling onto their face.

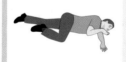

4 The recovery position:
☐ Once in the recovery position, do not leave casualty unattended, and continue to check breathing and pulse regularly.

KEY POINT
Even if you are not the appointed person at work who is responsible for dealing with first aid emergencies, it is important to have some basic training. As you will be working with members of the public we strongly urge you to complete a recognised three-day training course. Recognised courses are available through the British Red Cross (Telephone 0870 170 9110) and St. John Ambulance (0870 010 4950).

The first aid kit

There is no standard list of items which should be included in a first aid kit, but the Health and Safety Executive recommends the following as a minimum:

☐ **A guidance card or leaflet** which gives basic information about the most important emergency procedures

☐ **20 individually wrapped sterile adhesive dressings** (plasters in assorted sizes) which can be used for protecting cuts and other breaks in the skin

☐ **2 sterile eye pads** which can be used to cover the eye(s) following eye injuries

☐ **4 individually wrapped triangular bandages** (preferably sterile) which can be used as (1) a pad to stop bleeding; (2) as a sterile covering for large injuries such as burns or scalds; (3) as a bandage; (4) as a sling

☐ **6 safety pins** which can used to secure bandages

☐ **6 medium wound dressings** (a sterile, unmedicated dressing pad with a bandage attached, size no 8 – approx 12 cm x 12 cm) which can be used to cover medium cuts and wounds

☐ **2 large wound dressings** (a sterile, unmedicated dressing pad with a bandage attached, size no 9 – approx 18 cm x 18 cm) which can be used to cover large cuts and wounds

☐ **1 pair disposable gloves** to be worn at all times when dealing with blood or other body fluids

☐ **IMPORTANT NOTE:** A first aid kit should not contain medication of any kind such as over the counter pain killers and/or anti-inflammatories.

The accident book

Every business which has ten or more people working in it is legally required to keep an accident book in which all accidents, no matter how small, are carefully recorded.

Even in smaller businesses it is a good idea to keep a note of any accidents involving yourself, your clients or your work colleagues, as you may need to provide details in the event of an insurance claim.

The accident book should contain details of:

☐ the date and time of the accident

☐ the nature of the accident, including where it happened

☐ a short description of any action taken, e.g. ambulance called and client taken to hospital; or cold compress applied and client sent home in a taxi

☐ the signature of the person who is responsible for filling in the accident book.

Did you know?

If any business holds information about its customers and suppliers, either on paper (client record cards) or in electronic form (a computer data base) the business must comply with the requirements of the Data Protection Act 1998.

In addition, since October 2004, the Health and Safety Executive (HSE) now requires that all information relating to individual accidents and health and safety events at work must be recorded in an Accident Book which meets the requirements of the Data Protection Act 1998. Further information can be obtained from www.hsebooks.com/Books

Dealing with a fire at work

Your salon should be equipped with the correct kind of fire-fighting equipment. Fire extinguishers are available to deal with different kinds of fires.

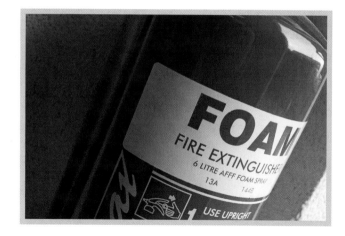
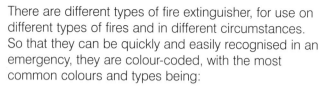
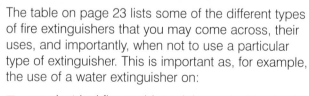

The extinguishers you have in the salon will depend on:

☐ the type of equipment used in your workplace

☐ how many treatment rooms there are

☐ how many clients, on average, visit the salon each day.

Your employer will provide the correct type and number of extinguishers, but it's vital that you know which type of extinguisher to use if you need to use one should a fire should break out.

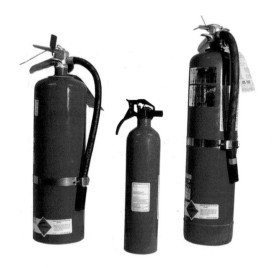

There are different types of fire extinguisher, for use on different types of fires and in different circumstances. So that they can be quickly and easily recognised in an emergency, they are colour-coded, with the most common colours and types being:

☐ Red (Water)

☐ Black (CO_2)

☐ Blue (Dry Powder)

☐ Cream (Foam).

The table on page 23 lists some of the different types of fire extinguishers that you may come across, their uses, and importantly, when not to use a particular type of extinguisher. This is important as, for example, the use of a water extinguisher on:

☐ an electrical fire could result in an electric shock

☐ a burning liquid fire could cause the burning liquid to explode.

Types of fire extinguisher

The types of extinguisher available, their recommended uses, and the colour-coding scheme may change from time to time, and you should keep up to date with current standards. The table on page 23 is adapted from www.fire.org.uk.

Type	Colour	Uses	Warnings
Water	Red	Fires involving solids – wood, cloth, paper, plastics, coal.	Do not use on burning fat or oil or on electrical appliances
Multi-purpose dry powder	Blue	Fires involving solids – wood, cloth, paper, plastics, coal. Liquids such as grease, fats, oil, paint, petrol, but not on chip or fat pan fires.	Do not use on chip or fat pan fires. Safe on live electrical equipment, although does not penetrate the spaces in equipment easily, and the fire may re-ignite. Does not cool the fire very well and care should be taken that the fire does not flare up again. Smouldering material in deep seated fires such as upholstery or bedding can cause the fire to start up again.
Standard dry powder	Blue	Liquids such as grease, fats, oil, paint, petrol, but not on chip or fat pan fires.	Do not use on chip or fat pan fires. Safe on live electrical equipment, although does not penetrate the spaces in equipment easily and the fire may re-ignite. Does not cool the fire very well and care should be taken that the fire does not re-ignite.
AFFF (Aqueous film-forming foam) (multi-purpose)	Cream	Fires involving solids – wood, cloth, paper, plastics, coal. Liquids such as grease, fats, oil, paint, petrol, but not on chip or fat pan fires.	Do not use on chip or fat pan fires.
Foam	Cream	Limited number of liquid fires.	Do not use on chip or fat pan fires. Check the instructions for suitability of use on other fires involving liquids. These extinguishers are generally not recommended for home use.
Carbon Dioxide (CO_2)	Black	Liquids such as grease, fats, oil, paint, petrol, but not on chip or fat pan fires.	Do not use on chip or fat pan fires. This type of extinguisher does not cool the fire very well and the fire may start up again. Fumes from CO_2 extinguishers can be harmful if used in confined spaces – ventilate the area well as soon as the fire has been controlled.
Fire blanket		Fires involving both solids and liquids. Good for small fires in clothing or chip pan fires if it completely covers the fire.	If the blanket does not completely cover the fire, it will not extinguish it.

Emergency procedures in the event of a fire at work

Employers are required, by law, to carry out a risk assessment, and to have a fire and evacuation procedure. By law, there must be at least one fire drill every year, which involves and includes everyone on the premises. Also, everyone must be fully informed and trained in what to do in the event of a fire.

You need to know:

☐ where the fire exits are in the building

☐ where the fire extinguishers are kept, and which kind of extinguisher to use for which kind of fire

☐ who to contact if you discover a fire, or if a fire breaks out where you are

☐ how to get your client safely out of the building

☐ where to gather – this is normally called the assembly point.

Sample building evacuation procedure

If you discover a fire has broken out:

☐ sound the alarm

☐ call 999 (112 within the EC) and ask for the fire brigade (better to be safe than sorry)

☐ if the fire is tiny and you feel confident that it can be safely, easily and quickly extinguished, use the appropriate fire extinguisher

☐ if you are at all unsure about whether or not you will be able to safely contain the fire with an extinguisher, your next priority is to get your client to safety

☐ if your client has undressed for their treatment make sure that they are provided with a robe and/or blankets and their own shoes.

☐ help your client to the nearest exit and take them to the designated assembly point

☐ wait at the assembly point with your client until the fire brigade arrives, and do not attempt to re-enter the building for any reason until you are told it is safe to do so.

END POINTS

By the end of this topic, you should understand that:

☐ your employer has a legal responsibility to provide a safe and healthy workplace, and safe equipment, working practices and procedures

☐ you have a legal responsibility to co-operate with your employer's health and safety policies and procedures, to work safely, not misuse any equipment or protective clothing that is provided and to take care of the health and safety of yourself, your work colleagues and clients

☐ it is vital that you know what to do in the event of either an accident or a fire at work

☐ a hazard is something that could cause harm – a faulty plug, a frayed carpet or broken stepladders

☐ a risk is the chance that a hazard will cause harm – a faulty electric kettle blows up and someone receives an electric shock; or a client catches their toe in a piece of frayed carpet and falls, breaking their ankle

☐ all accidents at work must be recorded in an accident book. The entry must be signed by both the person who filled in the details in the accident book and the person who was actually involved in the accident.

Topic 6: Safety, risk assessment and the salon

In the beauty salon, the main hazards to client and therapist include the:

- [ ] transmission of infectious diseases such as HIV or Hepatitis B
- [ ] use of chemicals
- [ ] safety of electrical equipment
- [ ] use of UV tanning equipment.

The next sections review some of the safety hazards that may be present in your salon, and suggest some ways of managing the risks they pose to staff and clients. This is not an exhaustive list, and will vary depending on the nature of your business and premises. The first step towards safety is a risk assessment. To begin assessing the risks in your environment, use the checklist at the end of this topic, and refer to some of the supporting material listed.

Hygiene

There is risk of transmission of infection when using equipment and products on different clients.

Managing the risks

- [ ] Ensure 'hard' re-usable equipment such as tweezers and cuticle knives can be sterilised between use on clients.
- [ ] Remember that 'ultra-violet sterilisers' do not sterilise. Ultra violet light has sanitising properties only.
- [ ] Use disposable products where possible, e.g. sterile disposable needles for electrolysis and orange wood sticks for manicures, to avoid the need to sterilise equipment between treatments.
- [ ] Provide 'sharps' boxes for disposal of needles, blades, etc. These should be disposed of by a registered operator.
- [ ] Use techniques which prevent cross-contamination.
- [ ] Thoroughly cleanse brushes, sponges, towels, etc. between uses.

- [ ] Contact your local council as you may need to register with them if you are carrying out skin piercing treatments.

Electrolysis

Under the Local Government (Miscellaneous Provisions) Act 1982, beauty salons that offer electrolysis must register with their local authority and comply with relevant byelaws made under the Act.

Managing the risks

The key points are to:

- [ ] use suitable equipment
- [ ] follow recommended methods
- [ ] have good standards of personal and environmental hygiene
- [ ] ensure staff are well-trained
- [ ] record all skin piercing treatments.

Waxing

The important issue with waxing is preventing cross-infection.

Managing the risks

☐ Hot and warm wax used for depilation should never be filtered and reused.

☐ Application should be with disposable spatulas that are then discarded.

☐ Observe good personal hygiene at all times.

Hazardous substances

Some preparations and products used in salons may contain harmful substances that can cause skin or respiratory problems. Cleaning products can also be hazardous.

Managing the risks

☐ Make a list of all hazardous products used in the salon and obtain hazard data sheets from the manufacturers.

☐ Use the ECOSHH website at http://www.coshh-essentials.org.uk/ to carry out a COSHH assessment.

☐ Remember to include the risks from blood-borne viruses in your COSHH assessment.

☐ If you have a shower on the premises, include the risk of exposure to legionella bacteria from water

☐ Make sure you are using the safest products available and that they comply with the Cosmetic Products (Safety) Regulations.

☐ Assess all new products before use.

☐ Store and use all products in accordance with the manufacturer's instructions.

☐ Dispose of surplus/out of date stock according to the manufacturer's guidelines.

☐ If dermatitis or asthma is detected action should be taken to minimise the problem by using barrier creams and gloves, improving ventilation, etc.

☐ Staff should be trained in the safe use of chemicals.

Use of cosmetic products in salons

All cosmetic products used in salons must comply with the Cosmetic Products Regulations 1978 and when using such products you must:

☐ follow instructions carefully

☐ never mix products unless recommended by the manufacturer

☐ keep the original containers and ensure all containers are properly labelled

☐ maintain good standards of 'housekeeping' and personal hygiene

☐ use appropriate protective clothing

☐ not use them on clients with abrasions or irritated scalps

☐ store them in a dry place, at or below room temperature

☐ keep them away from naked flames (especially aerosols)

☐ dispose of unused mixtures and empty containers properly

☐ keep containers sealed when not in use.

For more guidance, contact the Hairdressing and Beauty Industry Authority at Oxford House, Sixth Avenue, Sky Business Park, Robin Hood Airport, Doncaster, DN9 3GG (tel: 0845 2 306080) or see their website www.habia.org for more details.

Asbestos

It is now illegal to use asbestos in the construction and refurbishment of premises, but much of that used in the past is still there.

While it is undamaged and undisturbed, there is little risk, but if it is disturbed or damaged asbestos fibres may be released into the air where they will be a danger to health if inhaled. The owners, occupiers or managers of non-domestic premises which may contain asbestos, have a legal duty to manage the risk or to cooperate with those who manage the risk.

Managing the risks
- Ensure an assessment is or has been carried out as to whether asbestos is or may be present in the premises and record the results.

- If an assessment shows asbestos is or may be present, the measures which are to be taken to manage the risk must be specified in a written plan.

Electrical equipment

There are many different electrical appliances in use in beauty salons, and they are subjected to considerable wear and tear. Their portability and their proximity to water can create potentially hazardous situations.

Managing the risks
Appropriate precautions include establishing and maintaining an electrical equipment register and test/checking system, performing regular visual checks, fitting protective devices (such as a residual current device) to circuits to which portable hand tools are connected and ensuring correct earth bonding of pipework. A safe salon will:

- ensure electrical installations are maintained in a safe condition, and the state of fixed electrical installations inspected, tested and recorded by a qualified person every year

- have a system for regularly checking portable electrical equipment and an effective way of marking faulty equipment and preventing its use until repaired

- test all earthed appliances at periodic intervals

- keep a maintenance record for electrical equipment

- fit 30ma residual current devices (RCDs) to the main fuse board or to all sockets that hand held equipment and sunbeds are connected to

- provide adequate sockets so that sockets are not overloaded through the use of adaptors

- ensure that all hot and cold water pipes are suitably bonded and earthed

- ensure that any mains gas pipework is suitably earthed.

Sunbeds and other ultra violet tanning equipment

Exposure to ultra violet light has associated health risks. A poorly-maintained sunbed may represent a risk of electric shock or fire. Precautions to manage risks will include the safe construction, installation and maintenance of the equipment, safe working practices that limit client exposure and the suitable training of therapists.

Managing the risks

☐ Make sure sunbeds have regular, recorded, services and maintenance and correct ventilation.

☐ Ensure sunbeds can be electrically isolated and there is an emergency cutout switch for the client's use.

☐ Ensure sunbeds have effective timers fitted, and that there is a way for the client to summon assistance in an emergency. In an emergency, the door of the sunbed room should be capable of being opened from the outside.

☐ Staff should understand the hazards associated with ultra violet light emitted by sunbeds and how to control their exposure to it.

☐ Potential customers should complete a medical questionnaire before their first session.

☐ Keep clients' records, advise them of the health risks and the precautions they should take when using sunbeds. Instruct them on how the sunbed operates, its safety features and the maximum duration and number of visits they can make each year. Place advisory notices about safety and exposure in the sunbed room.

☐ When bulbs are replaced, make sure you inform clients to reduce exposure time and by how much.

☐ Provide washing facilities for use before the session.

☐ Provide suitable eye protection.

☐ Make sure that sunbeds and eye protection are thoroughly cleaned between uses.

☐ Introduce arrangements to deal with emergencies such as fainting.

Fire

Many beauty products, particularly aerosols, are highly flammable and potentially explosive. Obstructions in fire exits can prevent escape and fuel fires.

Managing the risks

☐ Make regular checks to ensure all escape routes and fire exits are clear.

☐ Store cosmetic products, particularly aerosols, at or below room temperature, in a dry atmosphere, and away from naked flames or sources of heat

☐ Do not use gas heaters with a naked flame.

☐ Switch off and unplug all electrical appliances at night.

☐ Make sure employees understand what to do in the event of a fire.

☐ Heaters should be suitably located and fitted with guards to protect children and clients' clothing.

Slips, trips and falls

These may be caused by trailing cables or spilt liquids – most accidents happen when staff trip on leads or uneven floors, or are trying to reach items on high shelves. These hazards should either be prevented, in the case of trailing cables, or rectified promptly, in the case of spilt liquids.

Managing the risks

☐ Fasten cables and leads securely.

☐ Route cables overhead if possible.

☐ Keep passageways, workstations and stairs clear.

☐ Clean up spilt products immediately.

☐ Provide adequate lighting.

☐ Provide appropriate step ladders to reach anything not accessible from the ground.

Manual handling risks

Lifting and moving heavy items or working in poorly-designed spaces may cause back injury or muscular strain, known as musculoskeletal disorders (MSDs). These are by far the most common occupational ill health problems in the UK, but:

- ☐ there are things that can be done to prevent MSDs
- ☐ the preventative measures are cost-effective
- ☐ all MSDs cannot be prevented, so prompt reporting and proper treatment are essential.

Managing the risks

The Manual Handling Operations Regulations 1992 establish a hierarchy of measures for dealing with risks from manual handling. These are to:

- ☐ avoid hazardous manual handling operations so far as reasonably practicable
- ☐ assess any hazardous manual handling operations that cannot be avoided
- ☐ reduce the risk of injury so far as reasonably practicable.

In the salon these can be addressed by:

- ☐ avoiding lifting items which are too heavy – use trolleys, lifts or other devices where possible.
- ☐ using proper lifting techniques.
- ☐ ensuring therapists have sufficient room to move around when working and provide chairs that can be adjusted to suit the client or therapist.

If there are risks to employees from manual handling, then a manual handling assessment should be carried out. The HSE provides a tool (called the MAC tool) to assist with this on their website
http://www.hse.gov.uk/msd/mac/

Safety and risk checklist for beauty salons

Use the checklist below to initiate your risk assessment for your workplace. Remember that risks apply to clients, staff and members of the public.

Check	Yes	No
Have you identified areas of hazardous activity in your premises?		
Have you carried out risk assessments for each of the hazardous activities?		
Have you carried out any assessments required under COSHH 1994?		
Do you minimise exposure to hazardous substances through good working practices, good ventilation and staff training?		
Have you taken steps to prevent hand dermatitis, including staff training and the use of suitable gloves/skincare treatments?		
Have you registered any relevant skin piercing with the local council?		
Do you meet standards specified in byelaws governing skin piercing?		
Are the methods used for waxing such as to prevent the spread of infection?		
Is equipment so maintained and used to prevent the spread of infection?		
Do you have a register of all electrical equipment used?		
Is electrical equipment subject to a system of user checks and periodic inspection/testing as appropriate and are records kept?		
Are appropriate protective devices in place in the fixed electrical system?		
Is there a system in place to ensure safety in the use of UV tanning equipment?		

Useful sources of information

The following may be useful references or sources of information
relating to safety in the salon.

A guide to hygienic skin piercing
Public Health Laboratory Service, Communicable Disease Surveillance Centre,
1 Colindale Avenue, London, NW9 5EQ.

A short guide to managing asbestos in premises INDG 223 (rev3) Reprinted 12/04 C2000
HSE website or HSE's information line 0870 154 5500

Blood-borne viruses in the workplace: Guidance for employers and employees INDG 342 07/01 C1500
HSE website or HSE's information line 0870 154 5500

Code of Practice for Hygiene in Salons and Clinics
The Federation of Holistic Therapists, 38A Portsmouth Road, Woolston,
Southampton, Hampshire SO19 9AD Tel: 01703 422695

Controlling health risks from the use of U/V Tanning Equipment Leaflet IND (G) 209
HSE website or HSE's information line 0870 154 5500

Health and Safety Implementation Pack for Hairdressers
Hairdressing and Beauty Industry Authority, 2nd Floor, Fraser House, Nether Hall Road, Doncaster,
South Yorkshire DN1 2PH, Tel: 01302 380000.

Legionnaires' disease – a guide for employers IAC27(rev2) 05/01 C500
HSE website or HSE's information line 0870 154 5500

Manual Handling Assessment Charts Leaflet (MAC) INDG 383 08/03 C1000
HSE website or HSE's information line 0870 154 5500

Safety in the Salon
Hairdressing and Beauty Industry Authority, Oxford House, Sixth Avenue,
Sky Business Park, Robin Hood Airport, Doncaster, DN9 3GG – Tel: 0845 230 6080

Topic 7: Professional record keeping

Why are client records important?

When you meet a client for the first time, it is important that you gain a clear picture of their health so you can identify which, if any, treatments are contraindicated, and also to determine what it is that the client is hoping to achieve.

For example, is the client suffering from work-related stress and hoping that their facial massage treatments will help them to relax and improve their sleep pattern? Or maybe, is the client reasonably fit and well, but hoping that a series of facials will help to improve their skin tone and restore skin elasticity?

CHECKLIST

The key benefits of keeping complete and accurate client records are:

☐ you know how to contact a client if you need to cancel or re-arrange an appointment, or if there something you need to discuss with them

☐ if there is a health emergency while the client is with you, you will know who to contact, e.g. their doctor or a relative

☐ filling in the client record card will help you to get to know the client and find out about their likes, dislikes and what they hope the treatment will achieve for them

☐ you will have a written record of the client's health and medical history so that you will know which treatments are contraindicated. You can also keep a record as to whether or not the client has received approval from their doctor to go ahead with treatment, if the client has a medical condition that renders this approval necessary.

☐ if you are unable to keep an appointment with one of your clients, a colleague will have access to all the information they need so they can treat the client appropriately

☐ you can keep notes relating to which treatments the client has received, the outcomes, and whether or not the client wants to repeat the treatment again in the future.

Types of record cards

Client record cards tend to vary slightly from salon to salon, depending on the preferences of the person who owns the business, but they generally contain more or less the same basic information.

An example record card

SALON NAME
Client Consultation Form – *Make-up*

Client Name: **Date:**
Address:

                                                     Profession:
e-mail: **Tel. No:** Day
                                                                  Eve

---

PERSONAL DETAILS
Age group: Under 20☐ 20–30☐ 30–40☐ 40–50☐ 50–60☐ 60+☐
Lifestyle: Active ☐ Sedentary☐
Last visit to the doctor:
GP Address:
No. of children (if applicable):   **Date of last period (if applicable):**

CONTRAINDICATIONS REQUIRING MEDICAL PERMISSION – in circumstances where medical permission cannot be obtained clients must give their informed consent in writing prior to treatment. *(select if/where appropriate):*

Medical oedema☐   Skin cancer☐
Nervous/Psychotic conditions☐   Slipped disc☐
Epilepsy☐   Undiagnosed pain☐
Recent operations affecting the area☐   Whiplash☐
Diabetes☐   When taking prescribed medication☐
Other:

CONTRAINDICTIONS THAT RESTRICT TREATMENT *(select if/where appropriate):*

Fever ☐   Scar tissue (2 years for major operation and 6
Contagious or infectious diseases ☐   months for a small scar) ☐
Diarrhoea and vomiting ☐   Sunburn ☐
Under the influence of recreational drugs or Hormonal implants ☐
alcohol ☐   Recent fractures (minimum 3 months) ☐
Skin allergies ☐   Sinusitis ☐
Eczema ☐   Neuralgia ☐
Trapped/Pinched nerve affecting the treatment Migraine/Headache ☐
area ☐   Hypersensitive skin ☐
Inflamed nerve ☐   Botox/dermal fillers (1 week following treatment)☐
Undiagnosed lumps and bumps ☐   Conjunctivitis ☐
Localised swelling ☐   Stye ☐
Inflammation ☐   Eye infection ☐
Cuts ☐   Watery eyes ☐
Bruises ☐   Hyper-keratosis ☐
Abrasions ☐   Any known allergies ☐

SKIN TEST *(select if/where appropriate):*

Moisture content:	Excellent☐	Good☐	Fair☐	Poor☐
Muscle tone:	Excellent☐	Good☐	Fair☐	Poor☐
Elasticity:	Excellent☐	Good☐	Fair☐	Poor☐
Sensitivity:	High☐	Medium☐	Low☐	
Skins healing ability:	Excellent☐	Good☐	Fair☐	Poor☐
Skin tone:	Fair☐	Medium☐	Dark☐	Olive☐
Circulation:	Good☐	Normal☐	Poor☐	
Pores:	Fine☐	Dilated☐	Comodones☐	Milia☐

Protecting yourself

In order to protect yourself against possible claims, make sure that you:

☐ always complete a record card for a new client

☐ update the card with appropriate details every time you provide a treatment for that client.

For some treatments the client will need to have an initial patch test to ensure that they are not allergic to any of the products used. It is vital that you record details of when the patch test was carried out, and the results. If, at some time in the future, the client complains about an allergic reaction you will have the results of the patch test so you can confirm that, at the time of the test, everything was fine.

Did you know?

You are entitled to refuse to treat a client if they refuse to take a patch test. This is because, even if the client is willing to sign a waiver which makes it clear that they are willing to have the treatment without the test, this still leaves you, as the therapist, liable to a claim against you if the treatment causes problems for the client. This is because, professionally, you are responsible for carrying out the test.

END POINTS

By the end of this topic, you should understand that:

☐ a new record card should be completed for each new client, and should be carefully updated with all the relevant information every time the client receives a treatment

☐ even if the client decides that it isn't necessary, or that they are willing to risk it, it is your responsibility to carry out a patch test where this is the normal routine for a treatment – for example eyelash or eyebrow tinting

☐ if you do not carry out a patch test and the client develops an allergic reaction to a product you have used you, as the therapist, could be liable to a claim against you.

Chapter 2:
The anatomy and physiology of the face, head and neck

In this chapter we'll be looking at:

Topic 1:
The skeletal system

Topic 2:
The muscular system

Topic 3:
The nervous system

Topic 4:
The circulatory system

Topic 5:
The lymphatic system

Topic 6:
The structure of the skin

Topic 7:
The functions of the skin

Topic 8:
The pathology of the skin

introduction

A good working knowledge of the underlying structure and function of the bones, muscles and physiological systems of the body will help you increase the benefits of the therapies you provide to your clients.

Here we will look at the systems of the body in general, and specifically at the face, head and neck. We will look at the muscular, skeletal and circulatory systems particular to the lower limbs, hands and feet in Chapter 5.

Topic 1: The skeletal system

The skeleton or skeletal system consists of the bones and the joints of the body. It is a hard framework of 206 bones that supports and protects the muscles and organs of the human body. The skeletal system is divided into two parts:

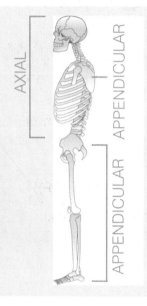

1. the axial skeleton: this supports the head, neck and trunk (also known as torso). It consists of the skull, the vertebral column, the ribs and the sternum.

2. the appendicular skeleton: this supports the appendages or limbs and attaches them to the rest of the body. It consists of the shoulder girdle, the upper limbs, the pelvic girdle and the lower limbs.

An easy way to remember the differences between the axial and appendicular parts of the skeleton is to think of axis (i.e. the centre) versus appendage (i.e. the added bits).

The centre is the head, neck and torso, the added bits are the arms and legs and the bones that attach them to the body. We will look at the appendicular skeleton in more detail in Chapter 5.

The structure and function of the skeleton

Structure

The skeleton is made up of bones. There are 206 individual bones in the human body and five different types, defined according to their shape:

1. **long bones:** the body's levers, they allow movement, particularly in the limbs e.g. the femur (thigh bone), tibia and fibula (lower leg bones), clavicle (collar bone), humerus (upper arm bone), the radius and the ulna (lower arm), metacarpals (hand bones), metatarsals (foot bones) and phalanges (finger and toe bones).

2. **short bones:** strong and compact bones, usually grouped in parts of the body where little movement is required e.g. tarsals (ankle bones) and carpals (wrist bones).

3. **flat bones:** protective bones with broad flat surfaces for muscle attachment e.g. occipital, parietal, frontal, nasal, vomer, lacrimal (all of these are in the skull), scapula (shoulder bone), innominate bones (pelvis), sternum (breastbone), ribs.

4. **irregular bones:** bones that do not fit into the above categories and have different characteristics e.g. vertebrae, including the sacrum and coccyx (backbone), maxilla, mandible, ethmoid, palatine, sphenoid, zygomatic (cheek) and temporal (all bones of the face and head).

5. **sesamoid bones:** bones within tendons. There are only two sesamoid bones in the human body, the kneecap, or patella, and the hyoid (base of the tongue).

The functions of the skeletal system

The skeletal system:

☐ supports the body: all body tissues (apart from cartilage and bone) are soft so without the skeleton the body would be jelly-like and could not stand up. The bones and their arrangement give the body its shape.

☐ allows and enables movement

☐ protects delicate body organs, e.g. the cranium, or skull, is a hard shell surrounding the soft brain, and the thoracic cage (ribs and sternum) covers the heart and lungs

☐ forms blood cells (in the red bone marrow)

☐ forms joints which are essential for the movement of the body

☐ provides attachment for muscles which move the joints: muscles are attached to bones and pull them into different positions, thus moving the body

☐ provides a store of calcium salts and phosphorus.

What are bones made of?

Bones are living tissue made from special cells called osteoblasts. The tissue varies considerably in density and compactness: the closer to the surface of the bone the more compact it is. Many bones have a central cavity containing marrow, a tissue which is the source of most of the cells of the blood and is also a site for the storage of fats. There are two main types of bone tissue:

1. **compact:** to the naked eye this looks like a solid structure but under a microscope it looks like honeycomb, i.e. full of holes. Haversian canals (see below) are passageways containing blood vessels, lymph capillaries and nerves which run through the tissue. Compact bone is found on the outside of most bones and in the shaft of long bones.

2. **cancellous:** this type of bone looks like a sponge and it is found at the ends of long bones and in irregular, flat and sesamoid bones. Bone marrow only exists in cancellous bone.

All bones have both types of tissue. The amount of each depends on the type of bone.

What are Haversian canals?

Haversian canals run lengthways through compact bone and contain blood and lymph capillaries and nerves. The larger the canal the less dense and compact the bones.

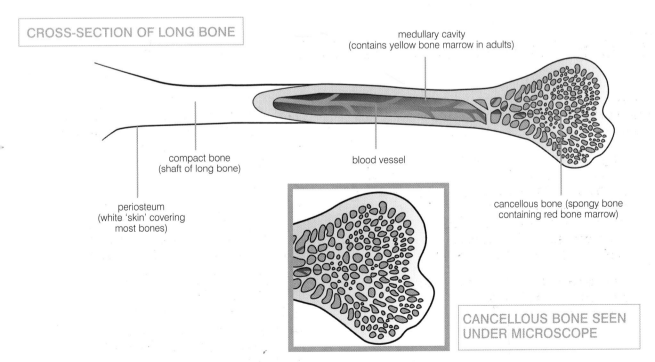

CROSS-SECTION OF LONG BONE

medullary cavity
(contains yellow bone marrow in adults)

compact bone
(shaft of long bone)

blood vessel

periosteum
(white 'skin' covering
most bones)

cancellous bone (spongy bone
containing red bone marrow)

CANCELLOUS BONE SEEN
UNDER MICROSCOPE

The axial skeleton

The axial skeleton includes the:

☐ **Skull:** cranium eight bones; face 14 bones,
hyoid: one bone

☐ **Vertebral column:** 33 vertebrae, some fused,
so 26 bones in total

☐ **Sternum:** three bones

☐ **Ribs:** 12 pairs (24 bones)

What is the skull?

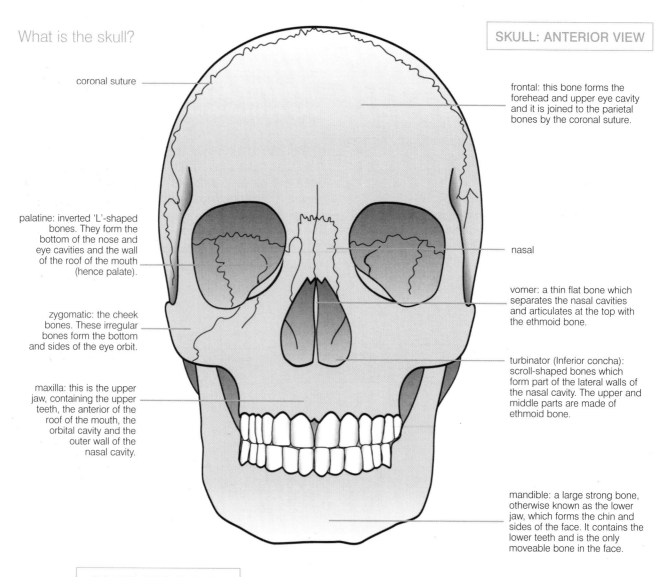

SKULL: ANTERIOR VIEW

coronal suture

frontal: this bone forms the forehead and upper eye cavity and it is joined to the parietal bones by the coronal suture.

palatine: inverted 'L'-shaped bones. They form the bottom of the nose and eye cavities and the wall of the roof of the mouth (hence palate).

nasal

vomer: a thin flat bone which separates the nasal cavities and articulates at the top with the ethmoid bone.

zygomatic: the cheek bones. These irregular bones form the bottom and sides of the eye orbit.

turbinator (Inferior concha): scroll-shaped bones which form part of the lateral walls of the nasal cavity. The upper and middle parts are made of ethmoid bone.

maxilla: this is the upper jaw, containing the upper teeth, the anterior of the roof of the mouth, the orbital cavity and the outer wall of the nasal cavity.

mandible: a large strong bone, otherwise known as the lower jaw, which forms the chin and sides of the face. It contains the lower teeth and is the only moveable bone in the face.

BONES OF THE FACE

SKULL: SIDE VIEW

lacrimal: very small bones positioned behind and lateral to the nasal bones. They are in the eye socket and contain foramina for the passage of the nasolacrimal duct (tear duct) hence their name.

ethmoid: the ethmoid is positioned below the frontal bone and in front of the sphenoid bone. It helps to form the orbital cavity (space for the eyes) and the nasal cavity (space for the nose).

nasal: two small bones which form the bridge of the nose. They articulate at the top with the frontal bone.

sphenoid: this bone forms the base of the cranium and it has wing-like projections (parts which stick out). It articulates with the frontal, parietal and temporal bones.

zygomatic

maxilla

mandible

coronal suture

parietal: these form the top and sides of the cranium.

occipital: this bone forms the back of the cranium. It has a large opening called the foramen magnus through which the upper part of the spinal cord passes. It articulates with the vertebra at the condyles of the skull.

temporal: these bones form the sides and lower part of the cranium; they are positioned below the cranium.

Hyoid (not pictured): V-shaped bone at root of tongue. provides attachment for muscles (i.e. tongue) and is the only bone not articulated with any other.

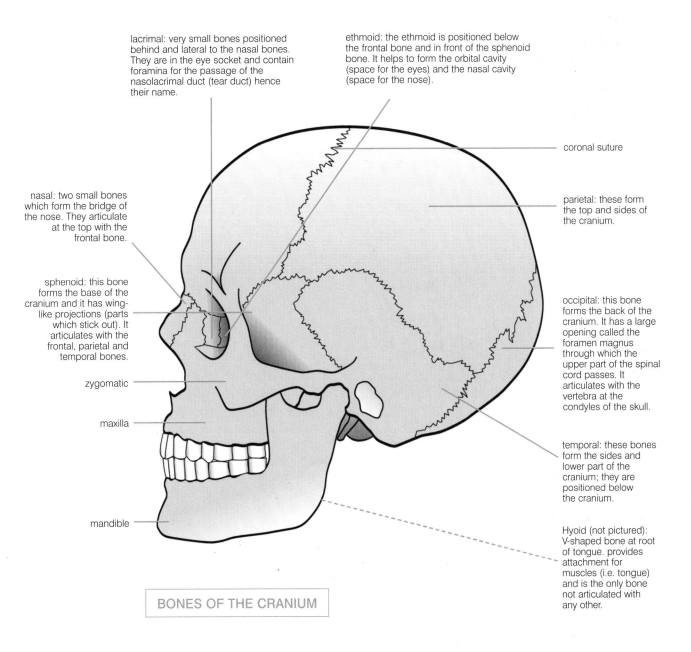

BONES OF THE CRANIUM

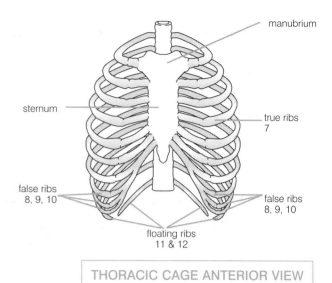

manubrium

sternum

true ribs
7

false ribs
8, 9, 10

false ribs
8, 9, 10

floating ribs
11 & 12

THORACIC CAGE ANTERIOR VIEW

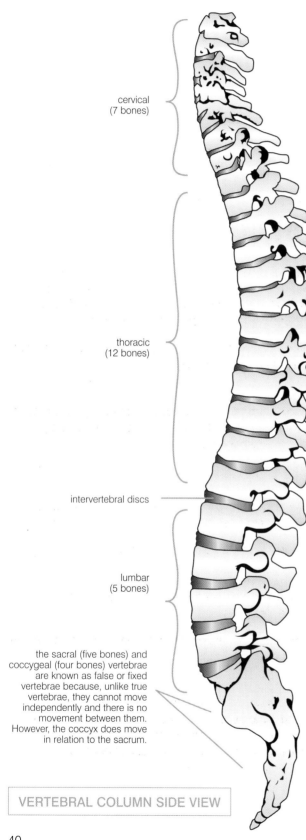

cervical
(7 bones)

thoracic
(12 bones)

intervertebral discs

lumbar
(5 bones)

the sacral (five bones) and coccygeal (four bones) vertebrae are known as false or fixed vertebrae because, unlike true vertebrae, they cannot move independently and there is no movement between them. However, the coccyx does move in relation to the sacrum.

VERTEBRAL COLUMN SIDE VIEW

The first three types of vertebrae are known as true vertebrae because they move. They are separated by intervertebral discs, pads of fibrocartilage, which have shock-absorbing functions.

What is the vertebral column?

A more common name for the vertebral column is the spine. It is the central part of the skeleton, supporting the head and enclosing the spinal cord and it is constructed to combine great strength with a moderate degree of mobility. It is made of 33 vertebrae — irregular, interlocking bones. Some of these are fused so there are only 26 individual bones. There are five different types of vertebrae:

1. cervical (7 bones in the neck)

2. thoracic (12 bones carrying the ribs in the centre of the body)

3. lumbar (5 bones in the lower back)

4. sacral (5 bones in the pelvis, fused to form the sacrum)

5. coccygeal (4 bones below the sacrum, forming the coccyx).

The joints

The joints are the hinges that join bones and enable movement of the limbs. There are three types:

1. fixed, or fibrous joints

2. slightly moveable, or cartilaginous joints

3. freely movable, or synovial joints

Diseases and disorders affecting the skeletal system

Arthritis

Arthritis is an inflammation of the joints. Mono-articular arthritis is an inflammation of one joint and poly-arthritis is an inflammation of many. It can be acute or chronic:

Acute: symptoms are heat, redness, and visible inflammation of the affected joints accompanied by severe pain.

Chronic: involves loss of cartilage, deposition of bone tissue around the joint margins and lesser degrees of pain and inflammation.

Gout

A form of arthritis that can occur in any part of the body but often affects the big toe; more common in men than women.

Cause: deposition of uric acid crystals within the joint capsule and cartilage.

Effect: attacks of acute gouty arthritis, chronic destruction of joints.

Osteo-arthritis (also known as degenerative)

Cause: may be injury of the joint or, if widespread, may be associated with the ageing process.

Effect: chronic arthritis of degenerative type – cartilage of joint breaks down; usually affects weight-bearing joints like knees, feet and back.

Rheumatoid arthritis (type of poly-arthritis)

Cause: an auto immune disease that attacks the synovial membranes and goes on to degrade and malform the articular surfaces of the bones.

Effect: acute and chronic phases with varying degrees of damage and deformity.

Ankylosing spondylitis

A type of arthritis with acute and chronic phases which results in fusion of the joints of the spine causing severe deformity and immobility.

Osteoporosis (also known as brittle bone disease)

Cause: calcium deficiency; accelerated bone loss especially in post-menopausal women.

Effect: porosity and brittleness of bones.

Slipped disc

Cause: the weakening or tearing of one of the intervertebral discs.

Effect: disc bulges or sticks out and this may press on the spinal nerve causing pain.

Stress

Stress is any factor which affects mental or physical health. When stressed, muscle tension increases and this causes poor posture (for example hunched shoulders or a clenched jaw), stiff joints and problems with the spinal vertebrae.

Interrelationships with other systems

The skeletal system links to the:

Muscular system: muscles always cross joints and thus rely on the framework of the skeleton for leverage and movement

Circulatory system: erythrocytes are produced in the bone marrow of long bones.

Nervous system: muscles require a nerve impulse to contract, which produces movement in the skeleton.

Digestive system: breaks down foodstuffs and works with the circulatory system to transport nutrients to bone tissues.

Urinary system: a hormone produced by the kidneys helps to stimulate the production of bone marrow in long bones.

ENDPOINTS

When you have finished this topic, you should know that the skeleton:

☐ is composed of bones and joints which form the axial (central head, neck and torso) skeleton and the appendicular (appendages – arms and legs) skeleton

☐ protects and supports the body, allows movement, produces blood cells (in red bone marrow), stores calcium and provides attachment for muscles

☐ is susceptible to breakage (fractures), and postural deformities caused by congenital or environmental factors.

You should understand the:

☐ structure of the skeleton including names and position of the bones

☐ function of the skeleton

☐ types of bone and bone tissue

☐ types of deformity, fracture and disease affecting the skeleton.

Topic 2:
The muscular system

Muscles are the body's movers and shakers. These tissues are attached to other parts of the body and when they relax and contract they enable movement. The muscular system is comprised of the muscles of the body and their attachments – tendons and fascia. When muscle fibres contract the muscles change shape and move whichever part of the body they are attached to. This can be a voluntary (conscious) movement such as lifting an arm or an involuntary movement such as vasoconstriction of the tiny muscles in the skin.

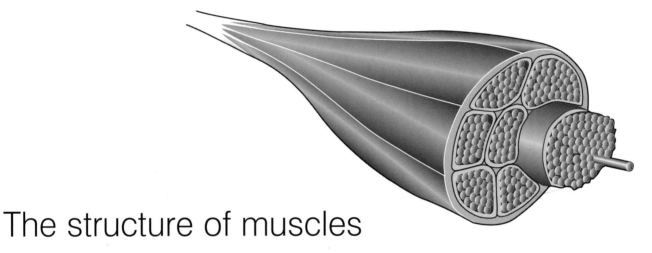

The structure of muscles

What is a muscle?
A muscle is a group of specialised, elastic tissues. More of the human body is made of muscle than any other tissue: 23% of a woman's body weight and about 40% of a man's.

Structure: muscle tissue is bound together in bundles and contained in a sheath (sometimes called a fascia), the end of which extends to form a tendon that attaches the muscle to other parts of the body. Muscle is 75% water, 20% proteins, 5% fats, mineral salts and glycogen.

Function: a muscle's function is to contract and by doing so start a movement in the surrounding structures (the tendons, ligaments and eventually bones). The muscle contracts in reaction to a nerve stimulus sent by the brain through a motor nerve. The muscle then shortens becoming fatter at the centre. In summary, the muscle's functions are to:

☐ contract and thereby produce movement, e.g. to move joints

☐ stabilise joints

☐ maintain postural tone

☐ aid in temperature control, e.g. shivering and dilation of capillaries (see Skin).

The smallest skeletal muscle (i.e. a muscle attached to a bone) is the stapedius in the ear. It activates the stapes, the stirrup-shaped bone in the middle ear which sends vibrations from the eardrum to the inner ear. The largest muscle in the body is the latissimus dorsi, the flat back muscle which covers the central and lower back. The strongest muscle in the body is the gluteus maximus which forms the main bulk of the buttock. This muscle is responsible for lifting the torso after bending down or leaning over.

What does muscle look like?

There are three types of muscular tissue, each with a different structure.

Voluntary muscle (sometimes called skeletal or striated muscle)

Function: these are the muscles which we consciously control e.g. our arms and legs – if we want to walk we do so.

Structure: voluntary muscle has cylindrical cells which make up fibres. Each fibre has several nuclei (multinucleated cells) and is surrounded by a sheath (sarcolemma).The muscle fibres form bundles and they all run in the same direction. Under a microscope voluntary muscle looks stripy. The stripes or striations are made of proteins (actin and myosin filaments) which run across the muscle fibres in transverse

bands; they are alternately light and dark and they give voluntary muscle its other name: striated muscle. When the muscle contracts the actin filaments slide between the myosin filaments, causing a shortening and thickening of the fibres.

Human babies, unlike some other mammals, are not born knowing how to control the voluntary muscles that help us stand and move. They learn to control and co-ordinate muscles in the following order: first the head, then the neck, the shoulders and arms, and then the lower parts of the body. When a baby finally learns to stand and walk, it has mastered all the muscles of movement because the last ones in the learning process are the pelvis and legs.

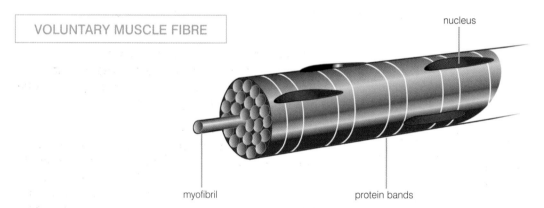

VOLUNTARY MUSCLE FIBRE

nucleus

myofibril

protein bands

Involuntary muscle (sometimes called smooth muscle)

Function: these are the muscles we do not consciously control, e.g. those that are found in the walls of blood and lymphatic vessels, in respiratory, digestive and genito-urinary systems. These muscles work automatically whether we want them to or not!

Structure: involuntary muscles have spindle-shaped cells with no distinct membrane and only one nucleus. Bundles of the fibres form the muscle we see with the naked eye. Under a microscope they have no stripes which is why they are also known as smooth muscles.

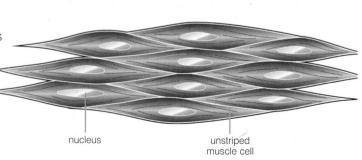

INVOLUNTARY (SMOOTH) MUSCLE

nucleus

unstriped muscle cell

Cardiac muscle

Function: to power the pump action of the heart.

Structure: cardiac muscle only exists in the heart; it is involuntary muscle tissue but its fibres are striated and each cell has one nucleus so, in structure, it resembles voluntary muscle. Each cell or fibre has a nucleus.

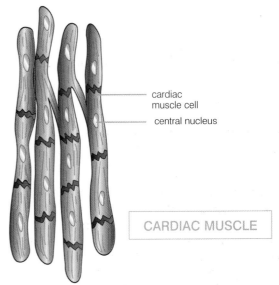

cardiac
muscle cell

central nucleus

CARDIAC MUSCLE

The functions of the muscular system

This section looks at how a muscle works and what we call its main components.

How do muscles work?

Muscles work by contraction: the fibres become shorter and thicker and the parts attached to the fibres (periosteum, bone, tendons and fascia) are pulled by the contraction and move. When a muscle fibre contracts it follows the 'all or nothing' law i.e. it contracts completely or not at all. Involuntary muscle and cardiac muscle contract independently of our conscious will. Voluntary muscles, however, move because we want them to, e.g. when we walk, lift our arm, hand or foot or bend down. There are two types of contraction:

1. **isometric:** the muscle contracts but produces no movement

2. **isotonic:** the muscle contracts and moves with the tension remaining unaltered within the muscle.

How does movement happen?

In skeletal muscles (those attached to bones) a muscle needs to pass over a joint to create movement. Muscle contraction pulls one bone towards another and thus moves the limb. Muscles never work alone: any movement results from the actions of several muscles. In general, muscles work in pairs. Each pair contains an antagonist (the opposing, relaxing muscle) and an agonist (the contracting muscle). The agonist and the antagonist must contract and relax equally to ensure a smooth and not jerky movement.

How does a muscle know when to contract?

The stimulus to contract comes from the nervous system through the nerves. Motor nerves enter the muscles and break into many nerve endings, each one of which stimulates a single muscle fibre.

Where does a muscle get energy from?

In order for contraction (and therefore movement) to take place, there must be an adequate blood supply to provide oxygen and nutrients and to remove waste products from energy production. Muscles receive their nutrients and oxygen from the arterial capillaries. This is converted into energy by chemical changes. The nutrients and oxygen are used up by the muscle and the waste product, lactic acid, is then excreted into the venous blood stream.

What affects a muscle's ability to contract?

A muscle's ability to contract is affected by:

☐ the energy available

☐ the strength of the stimulus from the nerve

☐ the time the muscle has been contracting

☐ an adequate blood supply bringing enough oxygen and nutrients

☐ the strength of the inhibitory nerve supply

☐ the temperature of muscle (warmth increases response)

☐ the presence of waste products like lactic acid.

Different stages of contraction

Tone: slight degree of contraction by some fibres as others are relaxing. In normal healthy muscles there will always be a few muscle fibres contracting at any one time, even during sleep. This action gives normal posture to the body.

Relaxation: a lessening of tension, so a reduction in the number of fibres contracting at any one time. Muscle tension can be affected by conscious effort and thought and relaxation can be taught.

Problems with over-contraction

Muscle tension: this is over-stimulation of muscle fibres. More fibres contract than are necessary to maintain postural tone.

Muscle fatigue: when stimulated, a muscle will need oxygen and fuel for its energy. This fuel is mainly glucose, stored in the muscle as glycogen and fats and transported by the blood. The muscle burns the glucose and fats by combining them with oxygen from the blood. Muscles that are repeatedly contracting and relaxing need a lot of energy and a lot of oxygen to produce that energy. That is why strenuous exercise causes rapid breathing and makes the exerciser out of breath.

If a muscle continues to contract without enough rest (e.g. if someone does too much exercise without breaks), the muscle will run out of oxygen and a by-product of this deficiency, lactic acid, will build up. This acid causes a burning sensation in the muscle, the muscle begins to quiver and soon stops contracting. The exerciser will feel stiffness and pain in the affected muscle. The muscle will not work properly until it can remove the lactic acid. It will need a fresh supply of oxygen for this. The exerciser will thus have to slow down.

Terms of description for muscles –

The names of the main components of a muscle system are show on the diagram on the opposite page. They are the:

☐ **attachment:** muscles can be attached by muscle fibres, tendons or other fibrous bands to each other, or to bones, skin, cartilage or ligaments.

☐ **belly:** thickest part or main body of muscle; usually the middle part away from insertion and origin.

☐ **insertion:** the moving end of the muscle, the point to which the force of the muscle is directed.

☐ **origin:** the fixed end of a muscle. This end of the muscle barely moves during muscle action. A muscle always works from its insertion towards its origin.

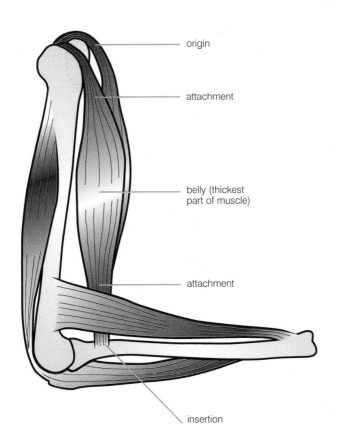

origin

attachment

belly (thickest
part of muscle)

attachment

insertion

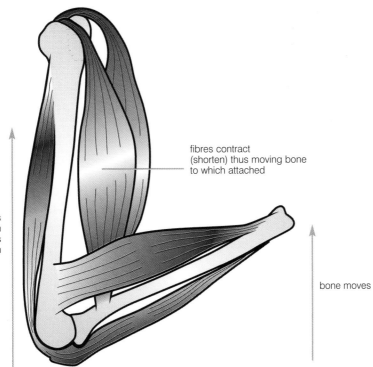

fibres contract
(shorten) thus moving bone
to which attached

muscle always
works from
insertion towards
its origin

bone moves

How are muscles attached to the rest of the body?

This section looks at the movement and position of the main muscles in the body. Muscles are attached to the rest of the body by tendons and the fascia.

Tendon

Structure: white fibrous cords (an extension of the fascia) with no elasticity which are of different lengths and thickness and are very strong. They have few, if any, blood vessels or nerves.

Function: it connects muscle to bone.

Fascia

Structure: white, fibrous connective tissue. It is found in all parts of the body, in different lengths and thicknesses.

Function: superficial fascia – beneath the skin; found over almost the whole surface of the body; facilitates the movement of the skin; serves as a medium for the passage of nerves and blood vessels; helps retain body warmth; connects skin with deep fascia.

Deep fascia – dense, inelastic, stiff membrane which forms a sheath (covering) for muscles and broad surfaces for attachment. Made of shiny tendinous fibres, it is thicker in unprotected areas and assists muscle action through tension and pressure.

Do all muscles work in the same way?

All muscles work by contraction but each muscle performs a specific action (type of movement) in order to move the body. There are several different actions:

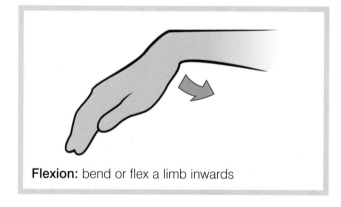

Flexion: bend or flex a limb inwards

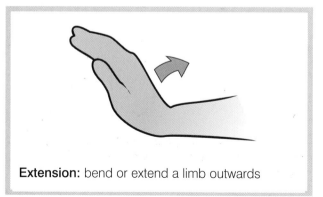

Extension: bend or extend a limb outwards

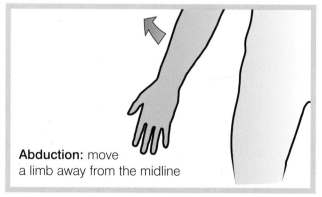

Abduction: move a limb away from the midline

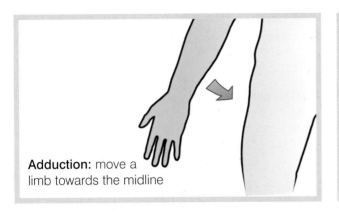

Adduction: move a limb towards the midline

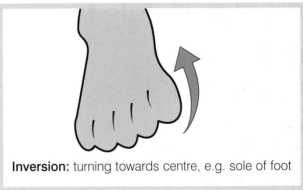

Inversion: turning towards centre, e.g. sole of foot

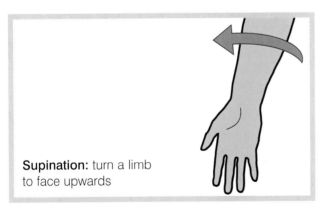

Rotation: rotate head at neck

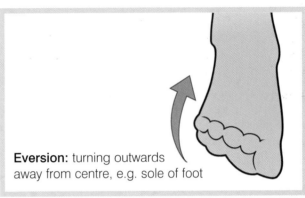

Eversion: turning outwards away from centre, e.g. sole of foot

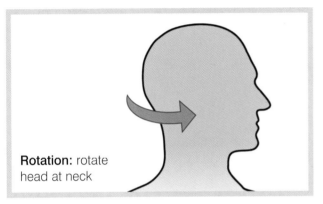

Supination: turn a limb to face upwards

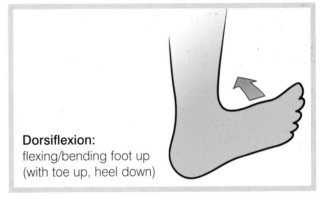

Dorsiflexion: flexing/bending foot up (with toe up, heel down)

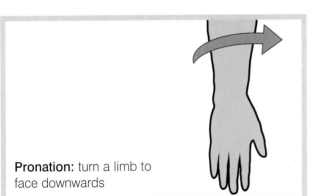

Pronation: turn a limb to face downwards

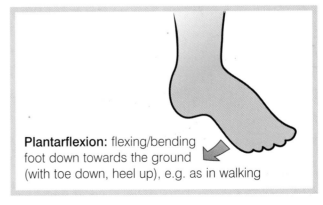

Plantarflexion: flexing/bending foot down towards the ground (with toe down, heel up), e.g. as in walking

The principal muscles of the head, neck and chest

There are thousands of muscles in the body. The diagrams in this section show the principal muscles of the body, detailing their position and their action.

MUSCLES OF THE FACE
(ANTERIOR VIEW)

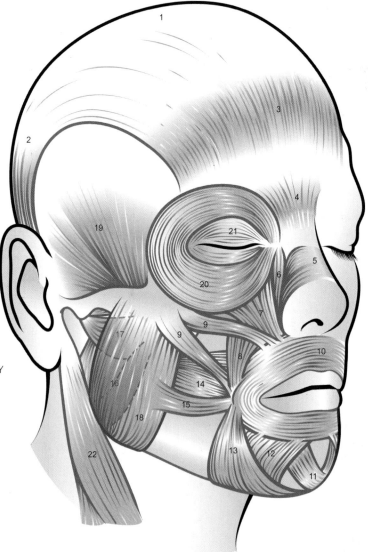

KEY: P: POSITION A: ACTION

1. OCCIPITOFRONTALIS
P: THE OCCIPITALIS AND FRONTALIS ARE COLLECTIVELY
   KNOWN AS OCCIPITOFRONTALIS
A: LIFTS EYEBROWS AND WRINKLES SKIN OF
   FOREHEAD; CREATES LOOKS OF SURPRISE
   AND HORROR

2. OCCIPITALIS
P: FIBROUS SHEET OVER OCCIPITAL BONE
A: MOVES SCALP BACKWARDS

3. FRONTALIS
P: FIBROUS SHEET OVER FRONTAL AND
   PARIETAL BONES
A: MOVES SCALP FORWARDS

4. PROCERUS
P: CONTINUATION OF FRONTALIS DOWN MIDLINE
   OF NOSE BETWEEN EYEBROWS
A: WRINKLES AT BRIDGE OF NOSE
   (DISGUSTED EXPRESSION)

5. NASALIS
P: SIDES OF THE NOSE
A: COMPRESSES AND DILATES NASAL OPENING
   (PRODUCES ANNOYED EXPRESSION AND SNIFFING)

KEY: P: POSITION   A: ACTION

6/7. LEVATOR LABII SUPERIORIS
P: THIN BAND OF MUSCLE FROM EYE TO MOUTH
A: LIFTS UPPER LIP; PRODUCES CHEERFUL EXPRESSION

8. LEVATOR ANGULI ORIS
P: THIN BAND OF MUSCLE BELOW LEVATOR LABII SUPERIORIS
A: RAISES CORNER OF MOUTH; PRODUCES CHEERFUL EXPRESSION

9. ZYGOMATICUS
P: THIN MUSCLE ANGLED ACROSS FACE SUPERFICIAL TO MASSETER
A: MOVES ANGLE OF MOUTH UP, BACK AND OUT (SMILING)

10. ORBICULARIS ORIS
P: SPHINCTER MUSCLE AROUND MOUTH
A: PURSES LIPS

11. MENTALIS
P: ABOVE MENTAL TUBEROSITY ON CHIN
A: LIFTS SKIN ON CHIN AND TURNS LOWER LIP OUTWARDS

12. DEPRESSOR LABII INFERIORIS
P: MID-LINE OF CHIN TO LOWER LIP
A: PULLS LOWER LIP STRAIGHT DOWN

13. DEPRESSOR ANGULI ORIS
P: FROM MODIOLUS TO MANDIBLE
A: PULLS DOWN CORNERS OF MOUTH

14. BUCCINATOR
P: BROAD THIN MUSCLE DEEP TO MASSETER
A: COMPRESSES CHEEK AGAINST TEETH TO MAINTAIN TENSION; AIDS IN MASTICATION

15. RISORIUS
P: BETWEEN MASSETER AND CORNER OF MOUTH
A: RETRACTS ANGLE OF MOUTH AND LIFTS UPPER LIP (PRODUCES GRINNING EXPRESSION)

16. MEDIAL PTERYGOID
P: INNER SURFACE OF MANDIBLE
A: RAISES THE MANDIBLE

17. LATERAL PTERYGOID
P: BEHIND THE ZYGOMATIC ARCH (CHEEK BONE)
A: PUSHES MANDIBLE OUT AND OPENS MOUTH

18. MASSETER
P: FROM ZYGOMATIC ARCH TO MANDIBLE
A: RAISES LOWER JAW; CHIEF MUSCLE OF MASTICATION

19. TEMPORALIS
P: FROM TEMPORAL BONE TO MANDIBLE
A: RAISES AND RETRACTS LOWER JAW

20. ORBICULARIS OCULI
P: SPHINCTER MUSCLE AROUND EYE
A: CLOSES EYELID

21. STERNOCLEIDOMASTOID
P: ROPE-LIKE MUSCLE RUNNING AT AN ANGLE UP SIDES OF NECK
A: FLEXES HEAD AND TURNS FROM SIDE TO SIDE

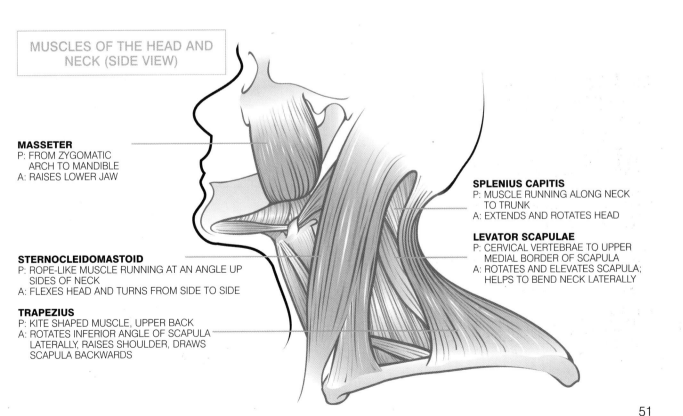

MUSCLES OF THE HEAD AND NECK (SIDE VIEW)

MASSETER
P: FROM ZYGOMATIC ARCH TO MANDIBLE
A: RAISES LOWER JAW

STERNOCLEIDOMASTOID
P: ROPE-LIKE MUSCLE RUNNING AT AN ANGLE UP SIDES OF NECK
A: FLEXES HEAD AND TURNS FROM SIDE TO SIDE

TRAPEZIUS
P: KITE SHAPED MUSCLE, UPPER BACK
A: ROTATES INFERIOR ANGLE OF SCAPULA LATERALLY, RAISES SHOULDER, DRAWS SCAPULA BACKWARDS

SPLENIUS CAPITIS
P: MUSCLE RUNNING ALONG NECK TO TRUNK
A: EXTENDS AND ROTATES HEAD

LEVATOR SCAPULAE
P: CERVICAL VERTEBRAE TO UPPER MEDIAL BORDER OF SCAPULA
A: ROTATES AND ELEVATES SCAPULA; HELPS TO BEND NECK LATERALLY

MUSCLES OF THE NECK, CHEST AND
ABDOMEN – ANTERIOR VIEW

KEY: P: POSITION A: ACTION

TRAPEZIUS
P: KITE SHAPED
   MUSCLE, UPPER
   BACK
A: ROTATES INFERIOR
   ANGLE OF SCAPULA
   LATERALLY, RAISES
   SHOULDER, DRAWS
   SCAPULA
   BACKWARDS

DELTOID
P: SHOULDER
A: FRONT DRAWS ARM
   FORWARD; MIDDLE
   ABDUCTS; BACK
   DRAWS ARM
   BACKWARDS

PLATYSMA
P: FRONT OF NECK
A: WRINKLES SKIN OF NECK

STERNOCLEIDOMASTOID
P: ROPE-LIKE MUSCLE
   RUNNING AT AN ANGLE UP
   SIDES OF NECK
A: FLEXES HEAD AND TURNS
   FROM SIDE TO SIDE

стена клайдомастойр

PECTORALIS MAJOR
P: CHEST
A: DRAWS ARM FORWARDS
   AND MEDIALLY; ADDUCTS
   AND ROTATES INWARDS

MUSCLES OF THE NECK, CHEST AND
ABDOMEN – POSTERIOR VIEW

KEY: P: POSITION A: ACTION

SUPERFICIAL MUSCLES

DEEP MUSCLES

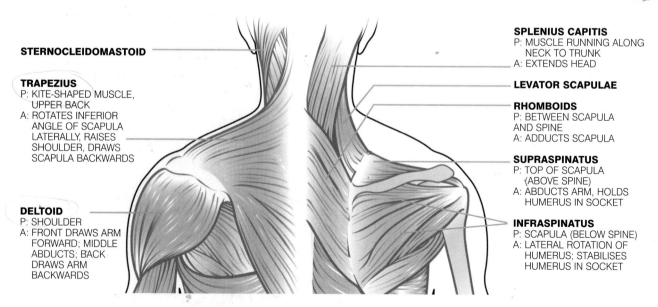

STERNOCLEIDOMASTOID

TRAPEZIUS
P: KITE-SHAPED MUSCLE,
   UPPER BACK
A: ROTATES INFERIOR
   ANGLE OF SCAPULA
   LATERALLY, RAISES
   SHOULDER, DRAWS
   SCAPULA BACKWARDS

DELTOID
P: SHOULDER
A: FRONT DRAWS ARM
   FORWARD; MIDDLE
   ABDUCTS; BACK
   DRAWS ARM
   BACKWARDS

SPLENIUS CAPITIS
P: MUSCLE RUNNING ALONG
   NECK TO TRUNK
A: EXTENDS HEAD

LEVATOR SCAPULAE

RHOMBOIDS
P: BETWEEN SCAPULA
   AND SPINE
A: ADDUCTS SCAPULA

SUPRASPINATUS
P: TOP OF SCAPULA
   (ABOVE SPINE)
A: ABDUCTS ARM, HOLDS
   HUMERUS IN SOCKET

INFRASPINATUS
P: SCAPULA (BELOW SPINE)
A: LATERAL ROTATION OF
   HUMERUS; STABILISES
   HUMERUS IN SOCKET

Diseases and disorders of the muscular system

Here are some of the common diseases and disorders that affect the muscular system

Fibrositis
Cause: build-up of lactic acid inside muscles.

Effect: inflammation of soft tissues and stiffness and pain. Lumbago – fibrositis of muscles in lumbar region of back; torticollis, known as 'wry neck' – fibrositis of the sterno-cleido mastoid muscle causes head to sit to one side.

Cramp
Cause: vigorous exercise and overexertion; also extreme heat; sodium and/or water depletion.

Effect: painful localised and involuntary contraction of one or more muscles.

Atony
Lack of normal tone or tension in a muscle.

Atrophy
Cause: malnourishment; lack of use.

Effect: wasting away, or failure to reach normal size, of bulk of muscle.

Myositis
Inflammation of a muscle.

Rupture
Burst or tear in the fascia or sheath surrounding muscles.

Spasm
A greater than usual number of muscle fibres in sustained contraction, usually in response to pain. Fibres contract for much longer than is usually necessary.

Spasticity
Cause: inhibitory nerves have been cut.

Effect: spinal reflexes cause sustained contraction.

Sprain
Cause: sudden twist or wrench of the joint's ligaments

Effect: an injury or damage to a joint; painful swelling of the joint; the most commonly sprained joint is the ankle (often called a 'twisted ankle'). A sprained ankle is usually caused by the joint 'turning over', thus putting all the body weight on the ankle.

Strain
Cause: overexertion, over-stretching, over-use; failure to warm up before strenuous activity, especially sport.

Effect: an injury to a muscle or its tendon; may occasionally involve rupture (tearing) of muscle fibres, muscle sheath or tendon.

Stress
Cause: stress is any factor which affects physical or mental well-being.

Effect: excessive muscle tension and subsequent muscle pain, especially in the back and neck.

Interrelationships with other body systems

The muscular system links to the:

Nervous system: relies upon nerve impulses to produce a contraction in the muscle. Without nerve stimulus movement would not be possible.

Skeletal system: muscles always cross a joint and thus rely on the skeletal system for leverage and movement.

Digestive system: nutrition/energy in the form of glucose is received from the digestive system. If it is not immediately used it is converted to glycogen and stored in the muscle fibres for energy production later.

Circulatory and respiratory systems: muscles receive oxygen from the vascular and respiratory system.

ENDPOINTS

At the end of this topic, you should know that:

☐ there are three types of muscle: voluntary, involuntary and cardiac

☐ there are two types of muscle attachment: tendon and fascia

☐ voluntary muscles have a variety of actions

☐ muscles work by contraction.

You should understand:

☐ the different types of muscular tissue and their functions

☐ the different types of muscular attachment

☐ the different actions performed by muscles

☐ how muscles contract

☐ how lactic acid is formed and how it affects muscles

☐ the position and action of the major muscles in the face, neck and head.

Topic 3:
The nervous system

The nervous system is a communication and instruction network. It is composed of the brain, spinal cord and the nerves. The nervous system informs the brain (sending messages at 290 km/h) about what is happening and thus protects the body. There are two parts:

1. the central nervous system

2. the peripheral nervous system.

The brain is the main unit and it is connected to the rest of the body by nerve cells which function as messengers, carrying information to, and instructions from the brain. They report back on pain, sensation and danger so that the body can respond and remain in what is known as homeostasis: a stable physiological state.

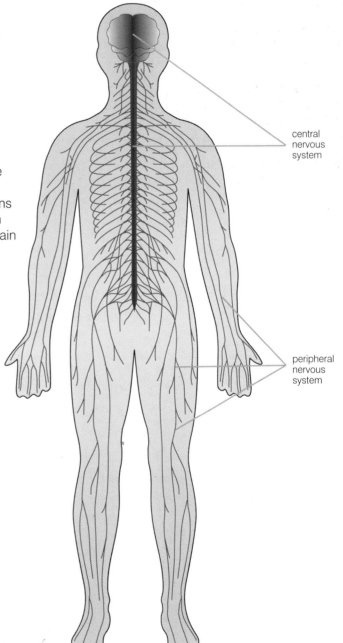

central nervous system

peripheral nervous system

Structure

What is the nervous system made of?

Nervous tissue which is composed of:

- [ ] nerve cells, known as neurones, with attached fibres

- [ ] neuroglia, a connective tissue which supports the neurones; though only found in the nervous system, neuroglia does not transmit nerve impulses.

What is a nerve cell?

Nerve cells are the basic unit of the system on which everything else is built. Like all cells, they have a membrane containing a nucleus and a cytoplasm but they have a particular shape: long and narrow. Some are very long (up to a metre).

Nerve cells are easily damaged by toxins and lack of oxygen. Unlike other cells in the body, they are not usually replaced when they die, however, current research suggests that some may have the ability to regenerate.

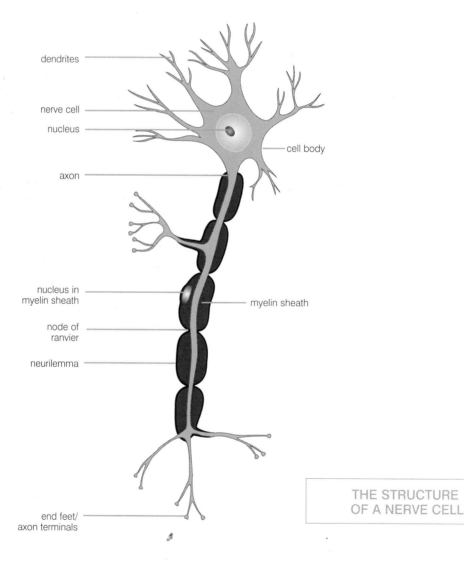

dendrites

nerve cell

nucleus

axon

cell body

nucleus in myelin sheath

myelin sheath

node of ranvier

neurilemma

end feet/ axon terminals

THE STRUCTURE OF A NERVE CELL

Function

What does a nerve cell do?

Nerve cells act as links in a chain, like relay runners, each one passing the 'baton' (information or instruction) to the next until it reaches the brain or the part of the body in question. The axon of one cell is close to the dendrite of the next but they don't actually touch. The 'baton' of nerve impulses jumps across the gap via neurotransmitters, chemicals released by the nerve endings.

Collective function

Individual neurones have the same function throughout the body, to transmit information, but collectively they make up five different types of nerves and nervous tissue which have specific functions:

☐ motor or efferent nerves: carry impulses from the brain or spinal cord to the muscles which then act on the information/instruction, producing movement or constricting a vessel. Motor nerves only transmit to glandular and muscular tissue.

☐ sensory or afferent nerves: carry impulses from all parts of the body to the brain.

☐ mixed: carry both motor and sensory nerve fibres. Mixed nerves are only present in the spinal nerves.

What is a nerve impulse?

Nerve cells transmit and receive impulses throughout the body. Nerve impulses do not continually run along each nerve. Impulses are created in response to particular stimuli, like changes in temperature, pressure or chemicals. These impulses are caused by chemical changes in the cell body. Chemical compounds generate electrical charges. Inside the cell there are potassium ions, which are positively charged, and the tissue fluid outside the cell contains sodium ions which are also positively charged. However, the membrane is more permeable to potassium than to sodium with the result that the outside of the cell has more positive charge than the inside. When there is a change of temperature or pressure, or a chemical reaction a section of the nerve membrane becomes permeable to sodium and the positively charged ions rush in, leaving the outside of the membrane negative. This reversal of polarity causes an electrical reaction which stimulates a change in the next section of membrane. The reaction continues the length of the nerve cell and this creates the impulse.

How do nerve cells communicate?

Nerve impulses only travel in one direction. So the movement of nerve impulses in a single neurone is as follows: the impulse crosses the synapse from the end feet of cell A into the dendrites of cell B. The impulse travels from the dendrites to the cell body and then out again along the axon to cell B's end feet. It then jumps across the synapse, helped by the chemical messengers. This process continues until the impulse reaches either the brain or the muscle/organ concerned.

The central nervous system

There are two parts to the nervous system in the human body:

1. central nervous system, consisting of the brain and spinal cord, both covered by meninges

2. peripheral nervous system, consisting of the cranial and spinal nerves and the autonomic nervous system which supplies nerves to all the body's internal organs.

The brain

The brain is the organ that fills the cranium (skull). It stops developing in the 15th year of life. It is the main mass exercising control over the body and mind and it has three different sections:

1. the cerebrum (also known as cerebral hemispheres)

2. the cerebellum

3. the brain stem.

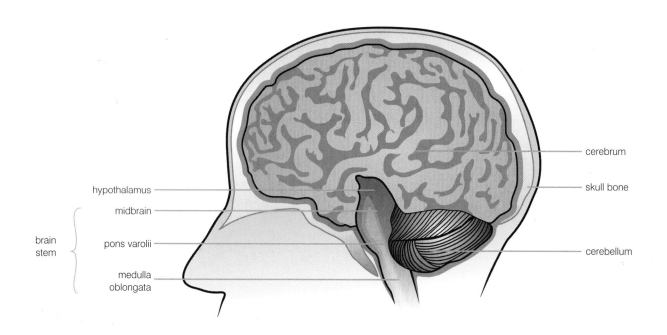

hypothalamus

midbrain

brain stem

pons varolii

medulla oblongata

cerebrum

skull bone

cerebellum

spinal cord

CENTRAL NERVOUS
SYSTEM – BRAIN

The peripheral nervous system

What is the peripheral nervous system?

The peripheral nervous system concerns all the nervous system outside the central nervous system and contains motor and sensory nerves which transmit information to and from the body and brain. It consists of 12 pairs of cranial nerves, 31 pairs of spinal nerves and the autonomic nervous system.

Cranial nerves

These nerves begin and end within the brain. They include the olfactory nerve, (the nerve of smell) and the optic nerve (the nerve of sight). The 12 pairs include motor, sensory and mixed nerves.

Spinal nerves

These pairs of nerves are divided into plexuses (groups of nerves which branch out to supply different parts of the body) named after the vertebrae to which they are connected:

- ☐ **cervical:** eight pairs
- ☐ **thoracic:** twelve pairs
- ☐ **lumbar:** five pairs
- ☐ **sacral:** five pairs
- ☐ **coccygeal:** one pair.

The lumbar, sacral and coccygeal nerves leave the spinal cord at the level of the first lumbar vertebra and extend downwards, forming a bundle of nerves known as the cauda equina (which means horse's tail in Latin, a reference to what the bundle looks like). These nerves group into plexuses with other adjacent nerves.

OPHTHALMIC BRANCH

FRONTAL nerve

LACRIMAL nerve

MAXILLARY BRANCH

INFRAORBITAL nerve

BUCCAl nerve

LINGUAL nerve

MANDIBULAR BRANCH

SUPRACLAVICULAR NERVE: 3RD/4TH CERVICAL

3RD CERVICAL (OCCIPITAL) NERVE

THE PERIPHERAL NERVOUS SYSTEM – THE CRANIAL NERVES

The autonomic nervous system

What is the autonomic nervous system?

The autonomic nervous system supplies nerves to all the internal organs of the body and to the blood vessels. It regulates events which are autonomic. It is controlled by the hypothalamus and its actions are thus not controlled by the brain or will, but are completely reflex and involuntary. Thus the brain does not know, and nor do we, when the actions happen. The system is divided into two parts:

1. sympathetic

2. parasympathetic.

Every organ in the body has a sympathetic and parasympathetic nerve supply.

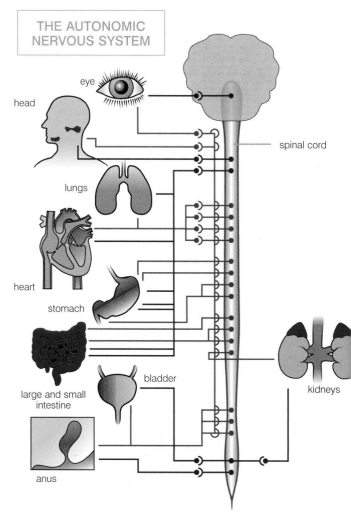

THE AUTONOMIC NERVOUS SYSTEM

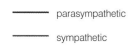
——— parasympathetic
——— sympathetic

Diseases and disorders of the nervous system

Neuritis

Inflammation of a nerve, caused by infection, injury, poison, etc.

Effect: pain along the nerve's length and/ or loss of use of the structures supplied by the nerve.

Bell's palsy

Facial paralysis, caused by injury to or infection of the facial nerve which subsequently becomes inflamed.

Neuralgia

Bouts of burning or stabbing pain, along the course of one or more nerves due to various causes.

Sciatica

Pain down the back and outside of the thigh, leg and foot, often caused by degeneration of intervertebral disc.

Parkinson's disease

Progressive disease caused by damage to basal ganglia of the brain and resulting in loss of dopamine (neuro-transmitter).

Effect: causes tremor and rigidity in muscles, as well as difficulty and slowness with voluntary movement.

Multiple sclerosis
Loss of the protective myelin sheath from nerve fibres in the central nervous system.

Effect: causes muscular weakness, loss of muscular coordination, problems with skin sensation, speech and vision.

Cerebral palsy
Damage to the brain, caused during birth or resulting from a pre-natal defect.

Effect: affects motor system control.

Motor neurone disease
A rare progressive disorder, in which the motor neurones in the body gradually deteriorate structurally and functionally.

Myalgic encephalomelitis (ME)
Known as post-viral fatigue. This disease is both difficult to diagnose and describe because the causes and effects differ. Symptoms include exhaustion, general aches and pains, headaches and dizziness.

Stress
Stress is any factor that affects mental or physical well-being. Emotions such as anxiety, fear and other negative feelings can affect the nervous system causing increased heart rate, breathing difficulties, sleep disturbances and stomach problems. All of these physical effects are caused by the nervous system over-working in response to stress.

Interrelationships

The nervous system links to:

All systems: nerves from the central nervous system control and receive information from every body system.

Muscular: muscles require a nerve impulse to contract.

Skeletal: muscle contraction (caused by nerve impulses) produces movement in the skeleton.

Circulatory: nerves control the heart rate.

Respiratory: nerves control the process of respiration.

Endocrine: works closely with the endocrine system to maintain homeostasis – balance in the body.

Skin: the skin contains a variety of nerve endings, at different levels in the layers.

ENDPOINTS
At the end of this topic, you should know that the nervous system has two parts, the central and peripheral (including autonomic) nervous systems, that it informs and warns the body of environmental changes, sensations, pain and danger and initiates responses to stimuli. You should also understand:

☐ the structure and function of the central nervous system

☐ the structure and function of the peripheral nervous system

☐ the structure and function of the autonomic nervous system

☐ what reflexes are.

Topic 4: The circulatory system

The circulatory or vascular system is composed of the blood, the heart, arteries and veins of the coronary, pulmonary, portal and systemic systems. Blood is pumped from the heart around the body through the transport system of arteries and veins. It distributes oxygen and essential nutrients to the whole body as well as removing potentially damaging waste products and carbon dioxide.

What is blood?

Blood is a fluid connective tissue made up of plasma and cells. Adult bodies contain approximately 4–5 litres whereas a new-born baby has only 300ml. It is alkaline (pH7.4).

What does blood do?
- [ ] transports oxygen, nutrients, hormones and enzymes around the body.

- [ ] transports waste materials from the body to the organs of excretion.

- [ ] helps fight infection (with leucocytes and antibodies – see opposite for more detail).

- [ ] prevents the loss of body fluids after accidents by clotting.

- [ ] regulates body temperature.

What is blood made of?
Blood is made up of plasma and cells

Plasma

Plasma makes up 55% of blood volume. It is a slightly thick, straw-coloured fluid. It is mostly water (90-92%) and the rest is plasma proteins (albumin, globulin, fibrinogen and prothrombin). Plasma helps to transport the following essential substances around the body:

- [ ] **mineral salts** – sodium chloride, commonly known as table salt, sodium carbonate and the salts of potassium, magnesium, phosphorus, calcium, iron, copper, iodine – which help nerve conduction and ensure that tissue cells keep the right acid balance.

- [ ] **nutrients** – amino acids, fatty acids, glucose, glycerol, vitamins. Most of these come from digested food and are absorbed (by the plasma proteins in blood) from the intestines to be used by cell tissues for energy, repair and cell reproduction.

- [ ] **waste** – waste products (like urea) are transported to the liver for breakdown, and then to the kidneys for excretion (eventually from the bladder as urine).

- [ ] **hormones** – chemical messengers produced by the endocrine glands. Plasma transports them to various organs and their job is then to change or influence that organ's activity or behaviour.

- [ ] **enzymes** – the chemical catalysts in the body. They produce or speed up chemical changes in other substances but remain unchanged themselves.

- [ ] **gases** – oxygen and CO_2 are dissolved in plasma.

- [ ] **antibodies and antitoxins** – the body's protectors. These complex proteins are produced in the lymph glands in response to the presence of toxins released by viruses and bacteria. Each antibody/antitoxin attacks a specific toxin (also known as antigen).

THE STRUCTURE OF BLOOD

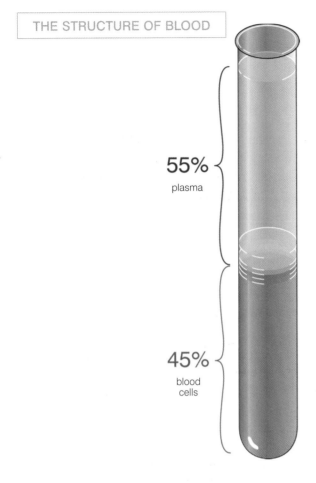

55%
plasma

45%
blood
cells

There are three types of blood cells – erythrocytes, leucocytes and thrombocytes.

Erythrocytes (also known as red corpuscles/blood cells)

Structure: biconcave, nucleus free discs

Function: transport oxygen as oxyhaemoglobin (for which iron and vitamin B12 are required).

General characteristics:

☐ produced in red bone marrow

☐ give blood its characteristic red colour, thanks to a protein called haemoglobin which absorbs oxygen

☐ life span of about 120 days

☐ broken down in the spleen and then the liver (where any spare iron is retrieved and recycled).

Leucocytes (also known as white corpuscles/blood cells)

There are two main types of leucocytes – granulocytes and non-granular leucocytes.

Structure: larger than erythrocytes, with an irregular shape and a nucleus

Function: to protect the body from infection.

General characteristics:

☐ approximately 8000 per mm^3 in a healthy body

☐ increase rapidly by mitosis in cases of serious infection.

Specific characteristics of granulocytes:

☐ defend system against microorganisms (e.g. viruses and bacteria)

☐ form 75% of white blood cells

☐ attracted by toxins into the tissues and can pass through capillary walls.

Specific characteristics of non-granular leucocytes:

☐ lymphocytes – some produce antibodies; formed in lymphatic tissue and found in all tissue except brain and spinal cord

☐ monocytes – eat bacteria and other micro-organisms (a process known as phagocytosis).

Thrombocytes (also known as platelets)

Structure: small, fragile cells with no nucleus

Function: responsible for blood clotting.

General characteristics:

☐ formed in red bone marrow

☐ 250 000 per mm^3 of blood.

The heart and systems of circulation

This section looks at how blood moves around the body, beginning with the heart.

The structure and function of the heart

How does blood circulate?

Blood is pumped from the heart (a muscular organ) around the body through a transport system of arteries, veins and capillaries. Pulmonary circulation is the transport of blood from the heart to the lungs and back again; systemic circulation is the transport of blood from the heart to the rest of the body and back. The blood circulation is two closed systems.

What is the heart?

The heart is the centre of the circulatory system (hence the use of the word heart to mean centre in English). If blood is the body's fuel, the heart is its engine.

What do arteries and veins do?

Arteries carry oxygenated blood from the heart and veins carry deoxygenated blood to the heart, except in the pulmonary system.

Arteries

Structure: arteries are thick-walled, hollow tubes. They all have the same basic construction:

- a fibrous outer covering

- a middle layer of muscle and elastic tissue

- an endothelial layer made of squamous epithelial tissue.

The quantity of muscle and elastic tissue in the middle layer depends on the size of the artery and its distance from the heart because arteries need to expand in order to propel blood along. Small arteries further from the heart have more muscle and less elastic tissue (because there is less blood to transport). The muscle tissue helps to maintain blood pressure and keeps blood moving around the body. The movement of the blood maintains potency (the openness of the vessel). Large arteries branch into small arteries which branch into arterioles which branch into capillaries.

Function: arteries (apart from the pulmonary artery) carry oxygenated blood from the heart to the body. The pulmonary artery carries deoxygenated blood to the lungs.

Arterioles

Structure: arterioles are a smaller version of arteries. They have a similar structure, though the middle layer of the walls is mainly involuntary muscle tissue (i.e. it has no control). This muscle is supplied with vasomotor nerves through which the vessel is contracted or relaxed. Under normal conditions all the arterioles are slightly contracted which helps to maintain blood pressure.

Functions: when a large blood supply is required by an active organ the arterioles relax and dilate to provide it (e.g. muscles during exercise, the stomach and intestines after eating and the skin when the body temperature rises). They contract when an organ is at rest.

General characteristics:

- the hormones adrenaline, noradrenaline and vasopressin (antidiuretic hormone) may cause the arterioles to contract

- in cases of shock, all the arterioles relax and blood pressure is very low. This is a dangerous condition.

Capillaries

Structure: capillaries are the smallest blood vessels. Their walls are one cell thick (i.e. microscopic) and porous, thus allowing the passage of gases (like oxygen and carbon dioxide) and nutrients. A large amount of water, plus the solutions dissolved in it, filters out through the capillary walls and bathes the body tissues. This liquid is called interstitial fluid. It carries food, vitamins, mineral salts and hormones out to the tissues and collects waste products, especially carbon dioxide and urea, from them. Most of the fluid then returns to the capillaries before they join up to become venules.

Function: to distribute essential oxygen and nutrients to most parts of the body. Capillaries supply every part of the body except the deep brain, the hyaline cartilage and the epidermis.

Venules

Structure: venules are small veins. These have a thin wall with a large passage (lumen) to carry the blood so they are easily collapsed under pressure.

Function: they carry deoxygenated blood from the capillaries to the larger veins.

Veins

Structure: veins have three-layered walls and, though the basic structure is similar to that of arteries, their walls are much thinner and the lumen (the passage in the centre which carries the blood) is much larger. They vary in size, the largest being the venae cavae (from the body into the heart) and the pulmonary vein (from the lungs to the heart). The action of skeletal muscles pushes blood through the vessels. Valves in the endothelial layer of the veins prevent a back flow of blood. Blood pressure in veins is very low so these valves are essential.

Function: veins carry deoxygenated blood back to the heart (apart from the pulmonary vein).

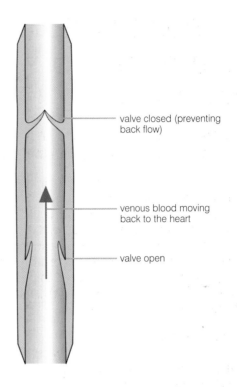

valve closed (preventing back flow)

venous blood moving back to the heart

valve open

This table summarises the different characteristics of arteries and veins.

Characteristics of arteries	Characteristics of veins
Transport blood from heart	Transport blood to the heart
Oxygenated blood (not pulmonary)	Deoxygenated blood (not pulmonary)
Lumen (passage) is small	Lumen (passage) is large
Pumped by heart and muscle tissue	Pumped by skeletal muscle pump and in artery wall the presence of valves
Thick, muscular and elastic walls	Thin walls, not muscular or elastic
Arterial blood contains a high concentration of nutrients	Venous blood contains a high concentration of waste products

Main arteries and veins of the body

The circulations begin at the heart. The inferior and superior vena cava bring venous blood into the right atrium, the pulmonary veins bring arterial blood into the left atrium.

The pulmonary arteries take blood to the lungs. The aorta, the main artery in the body, carries arterial blood to the body. It branches upwards to form the ascending aorta, which takes blood to the upper body (arms and head) and downwards, to form the descending aorta, taking blood to the rest of the body. Usually the names of veins correspond to the names of the arteries and they generally follow the same course, albeit in a different direction. When the blood reaches the various branches it is distributed through a network of arteries, arterioles and capillaries. The capillaries, the last vessels to distribute oxygenated blood, join the first vessels to collect deoxygenated blood, also called capillaries, which link up to form venules which feed into a network of veins taking the blood back to the heart for reoxygenation.

The following diagrams show the main veins and arteries that feed the face, head and neck.

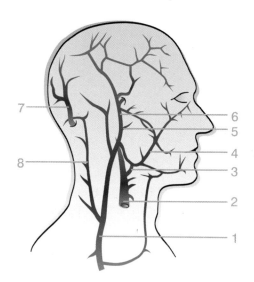

HEAD AND NECK
– MAIN ARTERIES

HEAD AND NECK
– MAIN VEINS

1. innominate artery
2. common carotid artery
3. internal carotid
4. external carotid
5. facial
6. occipital
7. superficial temporal

1. external jugular
2. internal jugular
3. common facial
4. anterior facial
5. maxillary
6. superficial temporal
7. occipital
8. posterior external jugular

Diseases and disorders

Varicose veins

Venous blood in the lower body has to move uphill in order to return to the heart. Valves prevent the blood flowing backwards but sometimes these valves, especially those in the superficial veins of the legs, no longer work effectively. Consequently the veins become dilated and blood collects in the veins instead of returning to the heart. The veins become distended and knobbly, showing through the skin. Varicose veins are often caused by:

☐ heredity
☐ excessive periods of sitting and standing
☐ pregnancy
☐ obesity.

Anaemia

Anaemia is a reduction in the blood's ability to carry oxygen, caused either by a decrease in red blood cells, or the haemoglobin they carry, or both. It may be caused by extensive loss of blood, lack of iron in the diet, the failure of bone marrow to produce the normal level of cells or it may be inherited.

Septicaemia

Also known as blood poisoning, this is a generalised disease associated with the circulation and multiplication of toxic bacteria in the blood.

Haemophilia

The blood's inability to clot. This is an inherited disease which affects mainly men but which can be carried by women.

Phlebitis

Inflammation of a vein. Thrombophlebitis is the inflammation of a vein where a blood clot has formed.

Thrombus

A blood clot in the heart or in the blood vessels.

HIV/AIDS

AIDS stands for Acquired Immune Deficiency Syndrome. It is a complex disease caused by the HIV (human immuno-deficiency) virus. The virus attacks T-lymphocytes, making the immune system incapable of fighting disease. It is transmitted through blood and other body fluids.

High blood pressure

Also known as hypertension, this is blood pressure which consistently remains above the normal level.

Low blood pressure

Also known as hypotension, this is blood pressure which consistently remains below the normal level.

Diabetes

A condition of the pancreas and the blood. Insulin (a substance produced in the pancreas) helps the body burn glucose for energy. If there is not enough insulin the blood contains too much sugar, fat is burnt instead and this is dangerous.

Hepatitis A, B and C

Inflammations of the liver, caused by viruses, toxic substances or immunological abnormalities. Type A is spread by fecally contaminated food. Types B and C are transmitted by infected body fluids including blood. Contagious.

Coronary thrombosis

A blood clot in the coronary artery.

Stress

Stress can be defined as any factor which affects mental or physical health. When a person is stressed, the heart beats faster, thus pumping blood more quickly. Excessive and unresolved stress can lead to high blood pressure, coronary thrombosis and heart attacks.

Interrelationships

The circulatory system links to other body systems:

Respiratory: carries oxygen to every cell and system of the body (internal respiration); removes waste gas from the body through diffusion between capillary/ alveoli (external respiration).

Lymphatic: linked to the lymphatic system at tissue level – the circulatory system transports some waste products away from the tissues (mainly carbon dioxide) and any additional waste products are carried away by the lymphatic system. The circulatory and lymphatic systems also work together to protect the body (immunity). The lymphatic system empties back into the blood system.

Endocrine: hormones carried in blood to various target organs.

Digestive: nutrients broken down in the digestive process are transported by blood from the small intestines to the liver then around the body.

Muscular: blood transports glucose for energy conversion to the muscles.

Urinary: blood passes through the kidneys for purification of toxins.

Skeletal: erythrocytes and leucocytes are manufactured in the bone marrow of long bones.

Skin: circulation transports oxygen and nutrition to skin, hair and nails.

ENDPOINTS

At the end of this topic, you should know that:

☐ blood is the body's fuel, delivered by the circulatory system, and it carries nutrients and oxygen to the body and collects waste and carbon dioxide from it

☐ the heart is the circulatory system's engine: it pumps blood around the body

☐ arteries and veins are the circulatory system's pipes.

You should know the:

☐ structure of the circulatory system

☐ function of the circulatory system

☐ position of the main arteries and veins in the face, neck and head

☐ diseases and disorders of the circulatory system.

Topic 5:
The lymphatic system

A circulatory system as complicated as that of the blood requires support. In the human body this is provided by the lymphatic system. The lymphatic system is a subsidiary circulation entwined with the blood circulation. It provides a channel through which excess tissue fluid is returned to the bloodstream.

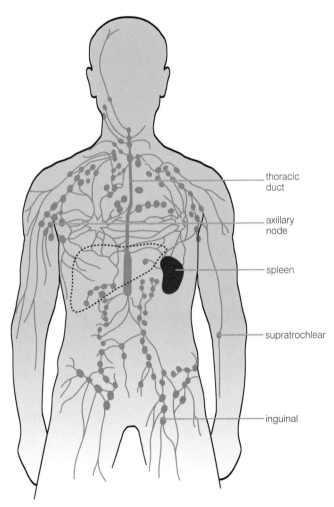

thoracic duct

axillary node

spleen

supratrochlear

inguinal

OVERVIEW OF THE LYMPHATIC SYSTEM
SHOWING LYMPH NODES AND SPLEEN

What is the lymphatic system?

In order to understand the lymphatic system it is necessary to understand what happens in the circulatory system at tissue level.

Blood travels to and from the tissues delivering nutrients and removing waste. Whole blood never leaves the capillaries, only its 'passengers' (i.e. oxygen, food, water) do and they are carried by a derivative of blood plasma called tissue, or interstitial fluid. This fluid circulates throughout the tissues, delivering food, oxygen and water to the cells and collecting carbon dioxide and other waste.

However, when it has finished its work and needs to return to the capillaries, not all of it can pass through the capillary walls because the pressure inside the capillaries is too high. The fluid that is left is picked up by a different set of capillaries, called the lymphatic capillaries. They have larger pores in their walls than blood capillaries and the pressure inside them is lower.

Thus, excess tissue fluid, substances made of large molecules, fragments of damaged cells and foreign matter such as micro-organisms drain away into them. The fluid, known as lymph, is filtered by the lymph nodes then collected by the lymphatic ducts before entering the right and left subclavian veins and returning to the bloodstream.

LYMPH CIRCUIT
(SIMPLIFIED)

lymph collects in ducts
before emptying into
the right and left
subclavian veins and
rejoining circulation

heart

lymph nodes filter tissue
fluid (lymph)

blood leaves
heart in
arteries and
travels to
tissues

blood returns
to heart in
veins

lymphatic capillaries collect
excess tissue fluid

tissue

What is the connection between blood and lymph?

The lymphatic system is a subsidiary circulation, helping
the blood circulation to carry out its functions.

It removes excess fluid from tissues and carries large particles that cannot pass through the smaller pores of the
blood capillaries. Lymph nodes and the spleen filter lymph (the name of the fluid in the lymphatic system) and
take out the waste materials it contains as well as producing antibodies and lymphocytes which are added to the
lymph to be transported to the blood.

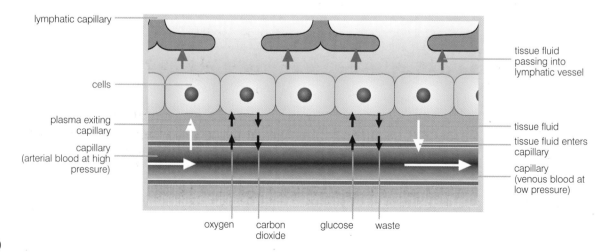

lymphatic capillary

tissue fluid
passing into
lymphatic vessel

cells

plasma exiting
capillary

tissue fluid

tissue fluid enters
capillary

capillary
(arterial blood at high
pressure)

capillary
(venous blood at
low pressure)

oxygen   carbon
          dioxide   glucose   waste

What is the structure of the lymphatic system?
The lymphatic system consists of lymphatic capillaries, lymphatic vessels, lymph nodes and lymphatic ducts. The fluid in lymphatic capillaries and vessels is called lymph.

What does it distribute and collect?
Lymph, a fluid similar to blood plasma.

Structure: contains waste materials as well as leucocytes and lymphocytes (in order to ingest bacteria and cell debris) but no erythrocytes.

Function: transports excess waste (that blood cannot carry) away from tissues; adds extra leucocytes and lymphocytes to the blood.

How does lymph move?
Several factors help to circulate lymph:

☐ the contraction of skeletal muscles collapses the vessels and because there are valves present, lymph is directed towards the upper part of the body

☐ a slight oncoming pressure from the tissue fluids

☐ movement of the lymph towards the thorax during inspiration

☐ suction: negative pressure helps to pull the lymph upwards into the lymphatic ducts, where lymph collects before being recirculated. These ducts empty into the subclavian veins which, because they are close to the heart, have negative pressure in them. This pressure pulls on the ducts and thus on the lymph vessels connected to them.

Any obstruction of the lymphatic flow results in oedema, the swelling of tissues due to the collection of excess fluid.

What are lymphatic capillaries?
The vessels which work with blood to collect excess tissue fluid. Lymphatic capillaries eventually unite to form lymphatic vessels.

Structure: fine, blind-ended permeable tubes, composed of a single layer of endothelial cells. They occur in all spaces between tissues, except in the central nervous system.

Function: carry excess tissue fluid away from tissue space.

What are lymphatic vessels?
These are vessels which transport lymph around the lymphatic system.

Structure: thin-walled, collapsible vessels similar to veins but carrying lymph not venous blood. They have valves (semi-lunar) to keep the lymph moving centripetally (in the direction of the heart) and prevent back flow. Consisting of a double layer of lining membrane, these valves give the vessels a knotted or beaded appearance. They have three layers:

☐ an outer layer of fibrous tissue

☐ a middle layer of muscular and elastic tissue

☐ an inner layer of endothelial cells.

Function: lymphatic vessels collect lymph from the lymphatic capillaries and then convey it towards the heart. Many lymph vessels run into the subcutaneous tissue (beneath the dermis) and all the lymphatic vessels pass through one or more lymphatic nodes.

What are lymph nodes?
All the small and medium-sized lymph vessels open into lymph nodes, which are strategically placed throughout the body. An afferent vessel transports lymph to the node and an efferent vessel transports the filtered lymph back to the system. Lymph nodes in the body are the:

☐ Submandibular nodes

☐ Deep and superficial cervical nodes

☐ Anterior auricular nodes

☐ Posterior auricular nodes

☐ Axillary nodes

☐ Supratrochlear nodes

☐ Inguinal nodes

☐ Popliteal nodes.

Structure: each node is made of lymphatic tissue, surrounded by a wall of tough, white fibrous tissue supported by inward strands of fibrous tissue called trabeculae. Lymph nodes vary in size.

Functions:

☐ to filter the lymph, remove and destroy harmful microorganisms, tumour cells, damaged or dead tissue cells, large protein molecules and toxic substances. This filtering system prevents toxic materials from reaching the bloodstream and causing septicaemia. If this occurs, it can cause the node to swell. In severe cases, this may cause cell destruction and an abscess on the node.

☐ to produce new lymphocytes and antibodies and add them to the lymph as necessary.

☐ lymphatic tissue cells within the node may become activated to form antibodies against a particular infection. They may then continue to form antibodies for several years or even a lifetime.

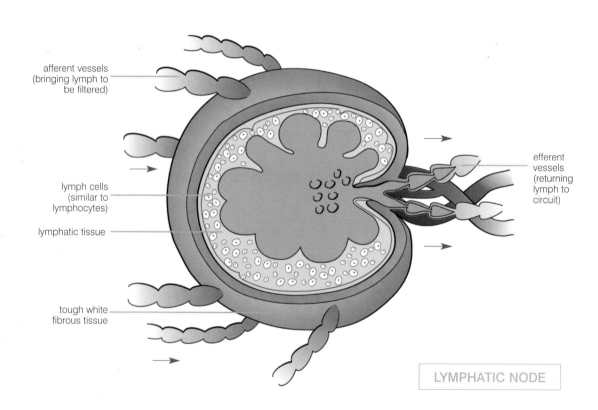

afferent vessels (bringing lymph to be filtered)

lymph cells (similar to lymphocytes)

lymphatic tissue

tough white fibrous tissue

efferent vessels (returning lymph to circuit)

LYMPHATIC NODE

Interrelationships

Lymphatic system links to:

- **Circulatory:** transports excess waste and toxins, which the circulatory system cannot cope with, away from the cells and tissues. Also works closely with the circulatory system to strengthen the body's immunity.

- **Digestive:** lymphatic vessels in the small intestines (inside the lacteal of the ileum) help with the absorption of fats during digestion. These are then transported around the body in the circulatory system and distributed to cells to be used as energy.

- **Muscular:** lactic acid formed when over-exercising muscles, or from tension and general fatigue in the muscular system, are drained away in the lymphatic system.

ENDPOINTS

You should now understand the structure, location and functions of the components of the lymphatic system, how it relates to other body systems, and that:

- it provides a channel for transporting excess tissue fluid away from tissues and back to the blood circulation

- it collects and transports lymph from tissue cells

- nodes filter lymph of harmful materials before returning it to the blood circulation

- it produces new lymphocytes

- it produces antibodies

- lymphatic capillaries in the lining of the small intestine assist in the absorption of fat droplets.

Topic 6:
The structure of the skin

The skin is the largest organ (group of tissues) in the body, both by weight and by surface area. It covers the whole body, is water-resistant, and has many functions including protecting and shaping the body. There are three layers: the epidermis, the dermis and the subcutaneous (hypodermis).

CROSS-SECTION OF SKIN

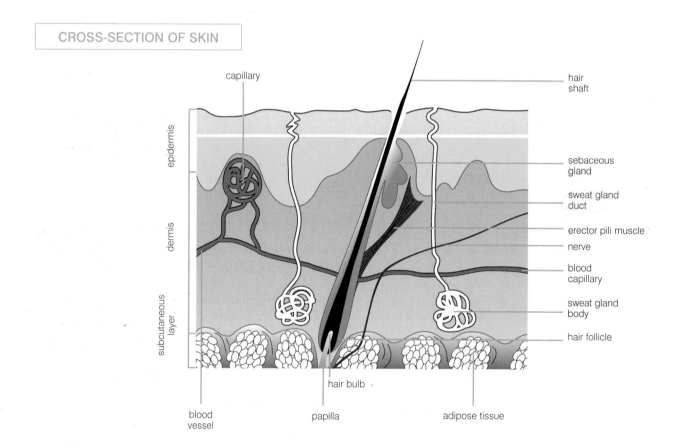

The epidermis

The epidermis is the layer of skin that we can see. It varies in thickness depending on the part of the body it covers.

It is thickest on the soles of the feet and palms of the hand and thinnest on eyelids. The cells on the surface are constantly coming off (this is called desquamation) and being replaced from below as cells in the basal layer of the epidermis multiply and are pushed up to the surface. There is no blood supply to the epidermis, hardly any nerve supply and it receives nutrients and fluids from the lymphatic vessels in the dermis.

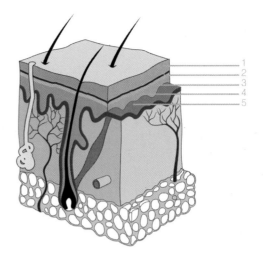

1. stratum corneum
2. stratum lucidum
3. stratum granulosum
4. stratum spinosum
5. stratum germinativum
   – basal

In total there are five layers in the epidermis:

1. Stratum corneum – the surface:

- is made up of hardened, flattened, dead, keratinised cells

- is constantly being shed through desquamation

- has an invisible cell membrane.

2. Stratum lucidum – clear layer:

- denucleated cells but not completely hard

- most easily visible under a microscope (only on palms and soles)

- cell membranes becoming visible.

3. Stratum granulosum – granular layer:

- cells have a distinct nucleus but cell membranes are dying

- contain granules which are visible in healing tissue after trauma.

4. Stratum spinosum – prickle cell layer:

- cells are living and membranes are intact; they have fibrils which interlock.

5. Stratum germinativum – basal layer:

- the primary site of cell division/reproduction (mitosis) in the skin

- cells are living. It is in this layer that cells are made. They take about 28–30 days to move up

from here through the five layers of the epidermis before being shed.

- this layer contains a pigment known as melanin that gives skin its natural colour, whether red, yellow or black. Melanin is produced by cells called melanocytes.

The dermis

The dermis is commonly known as the true skin. Unlike the epidermis, this layer is connected to the blood and lymph supply as well as the nerves. The dermis contains sweat and sebaceous glands, hair follicles and many living cells. It is made of connective tissue, mainly areolar tissue which is tough and elastic, and contains white collagen fibres and yellow elastic tissue known as elastin. Collagen plumps the skin and elastin keeps it supple and elastic. Both diminish with age. The dermis contains eight main types of structure:

1. Specialised cells

- fibroblasts: responsible for the production of areolar tissue, collagen and elastin. Fibroblasts can be damaged by ultraviolet light.

- mast cells: produce histamine as an allergic response and heparin, an anti-coagulant

- histiocytes: also produce histamine

- leucocytes: white blood cells which help to fight infection and disease.

2. Nerve endings:

- ☐ alert the brain and thus the body to heat, cold, pressure and pain
- ☐ part of the defence system of the body.

3. **Sweat glands** which stretch from deep in the dermis to the outer layer of the epidermis. Sweat contains mainly water, urea and salts (mostly sodium chloride), and is produced by two kinds of gland:

- ☐ eccrine: these excrete watery sweat and control body temperature, and are found all over the body, but especially on the palms of the hands and the soles of the feet.

- ☐ apocrine: these are found in the groin and axillae (armpits), and excrete a milky fluid which, when it mixes with bacteria on the surface of the skin, produces body odour.

4. Hair follicles:

- ☐ travel through the epidermis and the dermis.

- ☐ tiny muscles, called erector pili, are attached to each hair and help with the temperature control of the body by pulling the hair upright and trapping a layer of air – goose pimples.

5. Sebaceous glands:

- ☐ connected with hair follicles, and produce sebum, a fatty acid which keeps the skin moist and which lubricates the hair shaft. They are therefore found in hairy areas, not on the palms of the hands or soles of the feet.

- ☐ sweat and sebum combine on the surface of the skin to form the acid mantle, a protective shield which helps to control bacteria levels and prevents infections and disease and also acts as a natural moisturiser. The pH balance of the skin is 4.5–5.6 and this acid environment helps to prevent bacterial growth.

6. Blood supply:

- ☐ a system of blood vessels including microscopic capillaries which are one cell thick.

7. Lymphatic capillary:

- ☐ works in conjunction with the blood supply to carry waste products away from the area.

8. Papilla:

- ☐ small conical projections at the base of the hair

- ☐ contain blood vessels and nerves which supply the hair with nutrients.

The subcutaneous layer

This lies under the dermis and consists of a network of blood vessels, nerves, lymph and adipose tissue (fat cells). Its main function is to act as an insulator – both conserving the body's heat and acting as a shock absorber.

What are the component parts of a cell?

The diagram below is of a typical cell and the components, or organelles, which exist in different types of cell. It is meant as a guide, as cells may vary.

THE CELL AND ITS ORGANELLES

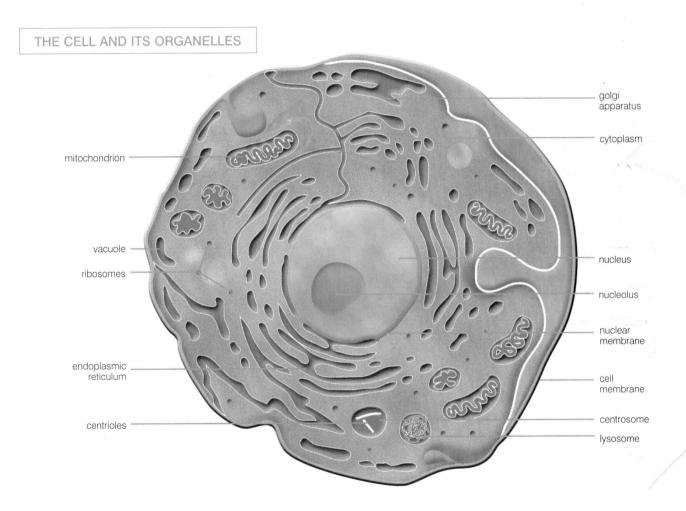

The components of the cell have different natures and functions.

Cell membrane

A fine membrane, made of protein threads and lipids (fats), which has two functions:

1. to keep the nucleus and the cytoplasm in the cell

2. to let other substances, like fats and proteins, out.

It works as a filter between the fluid inside the cell and the tissue fluid outside it. Some substances can cross this membrane but others are blocked. Substances go in and out of cells in several different ways:

- **diffusion:** the movement of substances from an area of high concentration to an area of lower concentration, depending on the difference in pressure on either side of the cell membrane.

- **osmosis:** the process of transferring water across the membrane by osmotic pressure – when the concentration or pressure of a solution is greater on one side of the membrane, water passes through to that side and vice versa until the concentration is equal on both sides. When both sides of the membrane have solutions of the same pressure, it is called isotonic pressure.

- **dissolution (or dissolving):** fatty substances are too big to diffuse through the membrane's tiny pores, so they dissolve into the fatty or lipid part of the membrane.

- **active transport:** when substances are too large to pass directly through the membrane, or are not soluble in fat, a carrier substance in the cell membrane takes them from the outside to the inside. Glucose and amino acids are both transferred by active transport. It is active because energy is used.

- **filtration:** the movement of water and soluble substances across a membrane caused by the difference in pressure either side of the membrane. The force of a fluid's weight pushes against a surface and the fluid is thus moved through the membrane. This is called hydrostatic pressure which is the process responsible for the formation of urine in the kidneys. Waste products are filtered out of the blood into the kidney tubules because of a difference in hydrostatic pressure.

Cytoplasm

Cytoplasm is the protoplasm inside the cell but outside the nucleus. It contains several different structures and substances.

Mitochondria

These organelles (little organs) are sometimes referred to as the 'power houses' of the cell, since they supply the cell with energy. Cell survival depends upon the chemical reactions that take place within the mitochondria, which result in a release of energy and the formation of ATP (adenosine triphosphate), the main energy transporter within the cell.

Endoplasmic reticulum

A network of membranes that forms a system of sacs and canals through the cytoplasm of a cell. It forms the circulation of the cell, allowing the movement of different substances.

Ribosomes

The 'protein factories' of a cell. They produce enzymes and other protein compounds; protein is used for the growth and repair of a cell.

Lysosomes

These organelles contain digestive enzymes which destroy worn-out parts of a cell and bacteria. They break down parts of food allowing them to be used for energy transfer within the cell.

Vacuoles

These are empty spaces within the cytoplasm. They contain waste materials or secretions formed by the cytoplasm and are used for storage or digestion purposes in different kinds of cells.

Golgi apparatus

The golgi apparatus combines polysaccharides (carbohydrates) with protein compounds and secretes these in order to send them to other parts of the cell for use as energy. It is a communication network from deep within the cell to its membrane.

Centrioles

These are paired, rod-like organelles that lie at right angles to each other. They are made of fine tubules which play an important role in mitosis (cell reproduction).

Centrosomes

Dense areas of cytoplasm containing the centrioles.

Nucleus

The very centre of the cell, the nucleus controls every organelle within the cytoplasm, and the processes of cell growth, repair and reproduction. It is contained within the nuclear membrane and its special protoplasm is called nucleoplasm. It contains DNA (deoxyribonucleic acid) which carries the cell's genetic code and chromatin, the material needed to form chromosomes. Chromosomes are made up of connected strands of DNA molecules, known as genes. A gene is therefore part of the length of a DNA molecule. Chromosomes carry inherited information which makes sure that when cells divide the 'daughter cells' are identical to the 'parent cells'. Each species is determined by the number of chromosomes in the nucleus. Human cells contain 46, i.e. 23 from each parent.

Chromatids

Two strands of chromatids held together by a centromere form a chromosome.

Centromere

The point where the two chromatids join in the chromosome.

Nucleolus

A small body within the nucleus that programmes the formation of ribosomes which then move into the cytoplasm of the cell and produce protein.

What does a cell do?

It lives! The human body is made of cells, which form organs, tissues, and fluid.

Blood, for example, is a liquid tissue made of several different types of cells. What a cell does is reproduced on a larger scale throughout the body and throughout human life: breathing, digesting, excreting, reproducing, sensing, growing, moving or, eventually, dying. When a cell goes wrong, the body goes wrong, since cell breakdown, and a subsequent inability to perform its usual functions, is the origin of disease and illness.

Cell functions include:

☐ Respiration: this is controlled absorption of oxygen that combines with nutrients in an oxidative reaction. This results in energy production and the formation of ATP. The waste produced is carbon dioxide.

☐ Growth: cells grow and repair themselves by making protein.

☐ Excretion: waste which might be harmful to the cell in large amounts, e.g. urea or carbon dioxide, is removed.

☐ Movement: whole cells, like blood cells, can move and parts of cells move, like the cilia of ciliated cells, but only in one direction.

☐ Reproduction: all cells grow to maturity and the majority then reproduce themselves. This can be simple cell division (mitosis) or sexual reproduction (meiosis).

☐ Metabolism: the chemical reactions that occur inside the cell.

☐ Anabolism: the chemical activity involved in the process of making new products (usually proteins) for growth and repair.

☐ Catabolism: the chemical activity involved in the breakdown of substances into simple forms, which results in the production of energy and waste. The energy is used to perform various cell functions.

☐ Sensitivity: cells are able to respond to stimuli, which can be mechanical, electrical, thermal or chemical.

How do cells grow/ reproduce?

Cells grow and reproduce through a process called mitosis. It is vital for living things to reproduce themselves in order to continue life.

Since the human body is made of cells, these cells must reproduce in order for the body to continue living. Mitosis is the multiplication of cells i.e. the constant process of making new cells in order for life to continue when the old cells die. This continues throughout life, except in the case of nerve cells, which are not always replaced when they die. Mitosis is faster in children and slows in later life. The process takes approximately two hours. If cells continue to divide and multiply they can create tumours and sometimes cancer. There are four stages of mitosis:

1 Prophase
☐ The centrosome divides into two centrioles. These move away from each other, though still joined by the spindle-like threads of the centrosome.

☐ Towards the end of the prophase the chromatin in the cell's nucleus shortens and thickens, forming into visible pairs of rods called chromosomes (made of condensed chromatin and DNA).

☐ Each chromosome consists of two chromatids joined by a centromere.

☐ The nucleolus disappears.

2 Metaphase
☐ The nuclear membrane of the nucleus disappears.

☐ The chromosomes arrange themselves at the centre of the cell, each attached to the spindle by its centromere.

☐ By the end of the metaphase, each individual chromosome can be seen distinctly as two chromatids starting to pull apart.

3 Anaphase
☐ The centromere stretches as the centrioles are drawn further apart.

☐ Pairs of chromatids divide and identical halves of the pairs move to each end of the cell.

☐ At the end of the anaphase, the spindle threads of the centrioles divide to form new centromeres and the cell membrane begins to constrict in the centre.

4 Telophase
☐ A new nuclear membrane appears around each set of chromosomes.

☐ The spindle fibres disintegrate and the centrioles replicate.

☐ The cell membrane continues to constrict until two cells are formed. These two daughter cells will be identical copies of the original single parent cell. Eventually, the daughter cells will also divide and the whole process continues throughout life.

5 Interphase
☐ The cell is resting.

☐ DNA is reproduced just before mitosis occurs.

☐ Nuclear protein is synthesised.

☐ Cell increases in size.

Meiosis
This is the cell reproduction which results in a gamete/sex cell. In meiosis, only half the numbers of chromosomes are present, 23 in the male sperm and 23 in the female ovum. When a male sperm fuses with a female ovum they create a zygote, a single complete cell with 46 chromosomes. The zygote will divide by mitosis and the organism that results from the cell division is called an embryo.

Did you know?
Inside a single, microscopic zygote, is all the information needed to make a new human

Cells and body tissue

As we saw, cells are the building blocks of our bodies. Many cells together make a piece of body tissue. There are four types of tissue: epithelial, connective, nervous and muscular.

Epithelial tissue (also known as epithelium)
There are two categories of epithelial tissue, simple and compound. Simple epithelium usually functions as a covering or lining for organs and vessels whereas compound provides external protection and internal elasticity. Goblet cells are often found in simple epithelium. These cells secrete mucus.

Simple epithelium

Simple epithelium consists of a single layer of cells attached to a basement membrane. There are four types: squamous or pavement, cuboidal, columnar and ciliated.

Squamous

Structure: single layer of flattened cells attached to a basement membrane

Function: forms a smooth lining for the heart, blood and lymph vessels and alveoli of the lungs.

Cuboidal

Structure: single layer of cubeshaped cells attached to a basement membrane.

Function: forms lining of kidney tubules as well as some glands; can secrete substances and absorb them.

Columnar

Structure: single layer of tall, rectangular cells attached to a basement membrane; resilient.

Function: forms lining in very active parts of the body such as the stomach, intestines and urethra; some of the cells secrete mucus and some absorb mucus, depending on where they are in the body.

Ciliated

Structure: single layer of mostly columnar cells (sometimes combined with squamous or cuboidal cells) attached to a basement membrane. Tiny hair-like projections, or cilia, stick out from the cell membrane.

Function: the cilia work in waves, all moving together in the same direction. They help to remove mucus, foreign matter and debris, keeping passageways and linings clear. The respiratory system is lined with these cells.

Compound epithelium

Compound epithelium has many layers of cells and no basement membrane. It is formed from a combination of deep layers of columnar cells plus flatter cells towards the surface. It protects delicate parts of the body. There are two types: stratified and transitional.

Stratified

☐ Keratinised (dry)

Structure: compound epithelium with dry surface cells;

forms a dead layer e.g. hair, skin, nails. It is keratinised (i.e. the surface layer has dried out into keratin, a fibrous protein which creates a waterproof layer). Skin is stratified, keratinised, squamous epithelium.

Function: the keratinisation prevents deeper layers from drying out and protects them.

☐ Non-keratinised (wet)

Structure: compound epithelium with wet surface cells e.g. inside mouth, lining of oesophagus, conjunctiva (mucous membrane) of eyes.

Function: provides lubrication.

Transitional

Structure: similar to stratified epithelium except that the surface cells are not flattened and thus can change shape when necessary; cube-shaped surface cells and deeper pear-shaped cells.

Function: found in organs that need waterproof and expandable lining e.g. bladder and ureters.

Nervous tissue

Structure: arranged in bundles of fibres, composed of nerve cells and neuroglia. The cells have long fibrous processes. On a nerve cell these processes are called dendrites and axons. Function: capable of transmitting signals to and from the brain; protective.

Muscular tissue

There are three types of muscle tissue:

☐ striated or voluntary

☐ smooth or involuntary

☐ cardiac.

Structure: all muscle is made of 75% water, 20% protein, 5% mineral salts, glycogen, glucose and fat.

Function:

skeletal: to help support and move the body;

smooth: to carry out involuntary functions, e.g. peristalsis;

cardiac: heart muscle to pump blood.

Connective tissue

Connective tissues are the supporting tissues of the body; they have mostly mechanical functions and connect more active tissues (like bones and muscles).

Structure: can be semi-solid, solid or liquid; can have fibres present or not.

Function: mainly mechanical connecting other more active tissues.

There are eight types:

1 Areolar

This is loose connective tissue, the most general connective tissue found in the human body.

Structure: semi-solid and permeable thus allowing fluids to pass through; it contains yellow elastic and white fibres as well as fibrocytes and mast cells which produce histamine (protection) and heparin (anti-coagulant, prevents clotting).

Function: found all over the body connecting and supporting other tissues e.g. under the skin, between muscles, supporting blood vessels and nerves and in the alimentary canal.

2 Adipose

This is also known as fatty tissue.

Structure: made up of fat cells containing fat globules; found between muscle fibres and, with areolar tissue, under the skin giving the body a smooth, continuous outline; also found around the kidneys and the back of the eyes.

Function: protective and insulatory properties: helps retain body heat because it is a poor conductor of heat; also a food reserve.

3 Lymphoid

Structure: semi-solid tissue; has some white fibres but not in bundles; lots of cells, the majority are lymphocytes and reticular cells which have a disease control function – the cell engulfs bacteria and destroys it.

Function: forms lymphatic system cells and blood cells and thus protects against disease; found in lymph nodes, thymus, the spleen, the tonsils, in the wall of the large intestine, the appendix and the glands of the small intestine.

4 Yellow elastic

Structure: mainly composed of elastic fibres and very few cells; this tissue is capable of considerable extension and recoil.

Function: to enable stretch and recoil e.g. forms lung tissue, bronchi and trachea, arteries especially the large ones, stomach, bladder and any other organs that need to stretch and recoil.

5 White fibrous

Structure: strongly connective but not very elastic; consists mainly of closely packed bundles of collagen fibres with only a few cells in rows between the fibres; the fibres run in the same direction.

Function: connection and protection of parts of the body e.g. forms ligaments and the periosteum of bone; forms the outer protection of organs e.g. around the kidneys, the dura of the brain, the fascia of muscles and the tendons.

6 Bone

Structure: hardest structure in the body; two types, compact and cancellous – compact is dense bone for strength, cancellous for structure bearing and cellular development; composition of bone is 25% water, 30% organic material, 45% inorganic salts.

Function: to support and protect the body and all its organs, as well as produce cells in bone marrow.

7 Blood

Structure: fluid connective tissue, containing 45% cells and 55% plasma. Cell content is erythrocytes (red blood cells), leucocytes (white blood cells) and thrombocytes (platelets).

Function: to transport food and oxygen to all the cells of the body and to remove waste from them

8 Cartilage

Structure: firm, tough tissue; solid and contains cells called chondrocytes. There are three types of cartilage:

Hyaline

Structure: bluish-white, smooth; chondrocyte cells are grouped together in nets in a solid matrix; particularly resilient.

Function: connecting and protecting; found on articular surfaces of joints i.e. the parts of bones that form joints; forms costal cartilages and parts of the larynx, trachea and bronchi.

Yellow elastic cartilage

Structure: yellow elastic fibres running through a solid matrix. Contains fibrocyte and chondrocyte cells which lie between multi-directional fibres.

Function: flexibility; found in parts of the body that need to move freely, like the pinna (the cartilaginous part of the ear) and the epiglottis.

White fibrocartilage

Structure: white fibres closely packed in dense masses; contains chondrocite cells; extremely tough and slightly flexible.

Function: to absorb shock, e.g. it forms intervertebral discs as well as the semi-lunar cartilages, the shock absorbers positioned between the articulating surfaces of the knee joint bones; also found in hip and shoulder joint sockets.

ENDPOINTS

At the end of this topic, you should know about:

☐   the structure of a cell

☐   the function of a cell

☐   mitosis – how cells reproduce

☐   meiosis – how humans are reproduced from cells

☐   the different tissue types made from cells.

Topic 7:
The functions of the skin

The functions of the skin

The skin has eight main functions:

1. Secretion: secretes sebum

2. Heat regulation: cools and warms body

3. Absorption: of drugs or essential oils

4. Protection: keeps out bacteria and creates barrier against rays of the sun

5. Elimination: of waste products

6. Sensation: skin is the organ of touch

7. Vitamin D production

8. Melanin production.

Secretion
The skin secretes sebum from the sebaceous glands. This fatty substance lubricates the hair shafts and when combined with perspiration on the surface of the skin, it creates a natural moisturiser which acts as a protective barrier against bacteria.

Heat regulation
Body temperature is maintained in healthy humans at 37°C (98.6°F). Organs involved in heat production are the muscles, liver and digestive organs. Heat is absorbed and maintained in the subcutaneous layer of adipose tissue. Heat regulation is controlled in the following ways:

Cooling
Vasodilation: when the body becomes hot, the capillaries dilate allowing more blood to reach the surface of the skin. The pores dilate allowing the heat to be lost from the body. This causes the skin to flush – this is known as hyperaemia. Sweating will occur simultaneously and the evaporation of perspiration from the surface has a cooling effect on the body.

Warming
Vasoconstriction: when cold, the body protects itself by moving blood from the extremities to the major organs, thus ensuring that they are kept warm. With the blood diverted to the deeper parts of the body, the capillaries contract as do the pores. As a result, the skin appears pale and heat loss is inhibited.

The erector pili muscles contract, causing body hair to stand on end, trapping air against the surface of the skin, which is then warmed by body heat. Shivering occurs, caused by rapid and repeated muscle contractions which work to raise body temperature.

Absorption
The skin is a waterproof covering but some chemical substances, such as drugs and essential oils, can penetrate the skin through the layers, the hair follicles and sweat glands. The amount of penetration is affected by the health and condition of the skin.

Protection
The skin acts as a barrier to the body's invasion by micro-organisms like bacteria. The naturally acid pH of the skin's surface inhibits bacterial production. Splits, cuts, tears and irregularities caused by disease or disorder increase the risk of infection. Melanin, the pigment produced by the melanocytes in the basal layer of the epidermis, has a protective function. It helps to protect against ultraviolet light damage to tissues. Sensory nerve endings found at differing levels in the dermis warn of possible trauma and, by reflex action, prevent greater damage to the body.

Elimination
Some toxins are eliminated from the body through the skin via the sweat glands. The toxins normally take the form of waste salts and water.

Sensation

Specialised nerve endings found in the dermis make the body aware of its surroundings. They warn of pain, cold, heat, pressure and touch. Different receptors lie at different levels in the skin. Pain and touch receptors are closer to the surface. All receptors warn of and help prevent trauma to the skin and underlying structures.

Vitamin D formation

Vitamin D is essential for the formation and maintenance of bone. Vitamin D production is stimulated by ultraviolet light which converts 7-dehydro-cholesterol in the sebum into vitamin D. This circulates in the blood and any excess is stored in the liver. Lack of Vitamin D can result in rickets in children.

Melanin formation

In the sun, the hormone MSH stimulates the melanocytes in the basal layer of the epidermis to produce melanin, a substance which produces a darkening of the skin to protect the underlying structures. The pigment protects the body from harmful effects of the sun's rays since dark colours absorb radiation.

ENDPOINTS

At the end of this topic, you should know the eight main functions of the skin.

Topic 8:
The pathology of the skin

As a major organ of the body, the one that is exposed to the elements and whose role is as an important line of defence for the body, the skin is susceptible to a range of diseases and disorders. These fall into six different categories:

1. Congenital (may be inherited), e.g. eczema

2. Bacterial, e.g. acne vulgaris

3. Viral, e.g. herpes simplex

4. Fungal, e.g. tinea pedis (Athlete's foot)

5. Pigmentation disorders, e.g. moles and freckles

6. General, e.g. comedones and milia (blackheads and whiteheads).

Congenital

There is a range of congenital (inherited) conditions that can affect the skin. These are some of the ones that you may come across.

Eczema: found all over the body but most often on the inside of the knee (in the popliteal space) and elbow joints, on the face, hands and scalp. The skin becomes extremely dry and itchy causing varying degrees of discomfort. Skin has scaly dry patches with bleeding at points. Not contagious.

Psoriasis: chronic inflammatory skin disease characterised by red patches covered with silvery scales that are constantly shed. Size of scales vary from minute spots to quite large sheets of skin. Points of bleeding may occur beneath scales. Affects whole body or specific areas, like face and scalp. Not infectious.

Bacterial

Acne vulgaris: normally caused by hormonal imbalances which increase sebum production leading to blocked glands and infection. The skin has a shiny, sallow appearance with papules, pustules and comedones. It is prone to open pores. Where pustules have cleared there is often pitting and scarring. The main sites for infection are the face, back, chest and shoulders. Not contagious.

Folliculitis: bacterial infection of the pilo-sebaceous duct (sebaceous gland and hair follicle) causing inflammation.

Boils: a bacterial infection of the skin, causing inflammation around a hair follicle.

Impetigo: a bacterial infection causing thin-roofed blisters which weep and leave a thick, yellow crust. Highly contagious.

Acne rosacea: gives a flushed, reddened appearance. Occurs on the face, this condition can be aggravated by anything causing vasodilation – heat, sunshine, spicy food, alcohol, cold. Affects both men and women especially menopausal women.

Viral

Warts: a small horny tumour found on the skin, often on fingers and thumbs. Caused by viral infection. Highly contagious.

Verrucas: warts found on the feet. Highly contagious.

Herpes simplex: a viral infection commonly known as cold sores; mainly found around the mouth. They appear as small blisters which, if left alone, will dry up leaving a crust which falls off. They are highly contagious when active.

Herpes zoster: a viral infection commonly known as shingles, which is the adult form of chicken pox, and usually affects spinal nerves and one side of the thorax. It is highly contagious.

Fungal

Tinea corporis, pedis: infections which attach themselves to keratinised structures like the skin. Tinea corporis is commonly known as ringworm and can be found anywhere on the body. Tinea pedis is commonly known as athlete's foot. Highly infectious.

Pigmentation disorders

Vitiligo: a complete loss of colour in well-defined areas of the face and limbs. A form of leucoderma (an abnormal whiteness of the skin due to absence of pigmentation); begins in patches but may converge to form fairly large areas; most obvious in darker skins.

Albinism: complete lack of melanocytes resulting in lack of pigmentation in skin, hair and eyes. Sufferers have poor eyesight and extreme ultraviolet sensitivity. This is an inherited condition.

Chloasma: butterfly mask often caused by pregnancy and the contraceptive pill; a pigmentation condition involving the upper cheeks, nose and occasionally forehead. Discolouration usually disappears spontaneously at the end of the pregnancy.

Ephelides: freckles; small pigmented areas of skin which become more evident on exposure to sunlight and are found in greatest abundance on the face, arms and legs; fair-skinned individuals suffer most from the condition.

Lentigo: also known as liver spots; dark patches of pigmentation which appear more distinct than freckles and have a slightly raised appearance and more scattered distribution.

Moles (papilloma): a common occurrence on the face and body and present in several different forms, varying in size, colour and vascular appearance. Flat moles are called sessile whilst those raised above the surface, or attached by a stalk are pedunculated.

Naevae: birth mark; if pigmented may occur on any part of the body and are often found on the neck and face, being sometimes associated with strong hair growth. Vary in size from pinhead to several centimetres and in rare cases may be extremely large. Pigmentation varies from light brown to black. Strawberry naevae (pink or red birth marks) often affect babies, eventually disappearing after a few years.

Port wine stain: a large area of dilated capillaries causing a pink to dark red skin colour which makes it contrast vividly with the surrounding skin. The stain is commonly found on the face.

General

Broken capillaries (couperose): dilated capillaries on a fine skin texture often affecting large areas of the face. The skin responds fiercely to stimulation and permanent dilated vessels are apparent, particularly on the upper cheeks and nose. Ruptured blood vessels assume a line-like appearance in surface tissues and can become bulbous and blue in colour due to the congestion in the blood vessels of the area.

Crow's feet: fine lines around the eyes caused by habitual expressions and daily movement, associated with ageing of muscle tissue. Premature formation may be due to eye strain and is often associated with oedema (swelling) around and under the eyes.

UV damage: UV rays stimulate rapid production of basal cells. This causes the stratum corneum to thicken. Over-exposure to UVA may cause premature ageing whereas over-exposure to UVB may cause skin cancer.

Urticaria – hives, nettle rash: often an allergic reaction. Characterised by weals or welts of pinkish colour produced by extreme dilation of capillaries. Very itchy. Can lead to secondary infection by bacteria through scratching.

Allergic reaction: when the skin is in contact with an irritant it produces histamine (part of the defence mechanism) in the skin. This can cause red, blotchy patches on skin, watery, stinging eyes, swellings and runny nose and can be slight or intense, depending on each person's reaction.

Comedones: commonly known as blackheads, these are caused by a build-up of sebaceous secretions which have become trapped in the hair follicles and have subsequently dried out and hardened. The colour comes from oxidation. Common in puberty.

Dermatitis: an allergic inflammation of the skin characterised by erythema – redness of the skin, itching and various skin lesions. Commonly known as contact dermatitis, there are many causes including plants, drugs, clothing, cosmetics and chemicals. Not contagious.

Milia: commonly known as whiteheads, these form when sebum becomes trapped in a blind duct with no surface opening. The condition is most common on dry skin and milia appear on the obicularis oculi muscle area and between the eyebrows.

Skin cancer

There are three main types of skin cancer, all caused by excessive exposure to sunlight:

Basal cell carcinoma

Occurs on exposed parts of the skin, especially face, nose, eyelid, cheek.

Squamous cell carcinoma

Squamous cells are those found on the surface of the body, in the top layer of the skin. Squamous cell carcinoma is said to be caused by sunlight, chemicals or physical irritants. It starts very small but grows rapidly, becoming raised.

Malignant melanoma

A malignant tumour of melanocytes. It usually develops in a previously benign mole. The mole becomes larger and darker, then ulcerated and the tumour eventually spreads.

ENDPOINTS
At the end of this topic, you should know the six categories of diseases of the skin.

Chapter 3:
Skin and eye treatments

introduction

Skin treatments are among the most common treatments performed by beauty therapists. A good working knowledge of the skin, how it works and possible dysfunctions, as well as an understanding of each client's skin, will form a solid foundation for the treatments you give, ensuring they will be safe and appropriate for each client.

Topic 1: Contraindications

Before you begin any skin treatments, you must be aware of all contraindications. Follow the guidelines in Chapter 1 for total contraindications, those needing GP or specialist permission and general localised contraindications, and always review the contraindications for a particular treatment before seeing a client. You should be particularly aware of all contraindications affecting the skin:

Contraindications requiring medical permission – in circumstances where medical permission cannot be obtained clients must give their informed consent in writing prior to the treatment

☐ Medical oedema	☐ Diabetes	☐ When taking prescribed medication
☐ Nervous/Psychotic conditions	☐ Skin cancer	
☐ Epilepsy	☐ Slipped disc	☐ Whiplash
☐ Recent facial operations affecting the area	☐ Undiagnosed pain	

Contraindications that restrict treatment

☐ Fever	☐ Cuts, bruises, abrasions	☐ Botox
☐ Contagious or infectious diseases	☐ Scar tissues (2 years for major operation and 6 months for a small scar)	☐ Dermal fillers (1 week following treatment)
☐ Under the influence of recreational drugs or alcohol	☐ Sunburn	☐ Hyper-keratosis
☐ Diarrhoea and vomiting	☐ Hormonal implants	☐ Skin allergies
☐ Any known allergies	☐ Recent fractures (minimum 3 months)	☐ Styes, watery eyes, eye infection, conjunctivitis
☐ Eczema	☐ Sinusitis	☐ Trapped/pinched nerve affecting the treatment area
☐ Undiagnosed lumps and bumps	☐ Neuralgia	☐ Inflamed nerve
☐ Localised swelling	☐ Migraine/Headache	
☐ Inflammation	☐ Hypersensitive skin	

ENDPOINTS

At the end of this topic, you should know the main contraindications to skin treatments, including those that:

☐ are subject to medical approval

☐ restrict treatment.

Topic 2: Skin analysis

Before carrying out skin treatments, it is important to take into account the client's skin type, colour and condition in order to choose the most effective and suitable treatments and the correct products. The skin analysis and consultation is when you begin to find out about your client's skin type and characteristics, and about any factors that might be affecting the skin's condition. The process of consultation may also be the first chance your client has to feel comfortable with your presence and technique, so it is a very important time to build up a good relationship with your client.

Methods for analysing skin type

A combination of methods is used to analyse the skin type

☐ consultation with the client (see Chapter 1 and below)

☐ initial visual check (see below)

☐ information already recorded on the client's record card, if an existing client (see Chapter 1 and below)

☐ feel of the client's skin texture and tone, and its reaction to initial cleansing treatment (see Topic 2)

☐ use of a magnifying lamp after initial cleansing (see below).

The analysis of the skin should determine:

☐ the client's skin type

☐ pigmentation and skin colour

☐ skin texture

☐ skin imperfections

☐ the tone of the skin

☐ the temperature of the skin.

Ageing of the skin

The signs of skin ageing generally appear as:

☐ a loss of tone in the facial expression muscles

☐ more prominent bones

☐ fine wrinkling around the eyes

☐ looser skin on the neck and eyelids

☐ generally finer and less elastic skin

☐ broken capillaries on cheeks and nose

☐ pigmentation becoming evident.

As well as the client's actual age, skin ageing is affected by:

☐ diet

☐ genetic factors

☐ exposure to sun, wind, pollution, etc.

☐ smoking and alcohol intake

☐ sleep patterns

☐ stress

☐ weight gain or weight loss

☐ general health and previous health problems

☐ general or specific skin care

☐ superficial hair.

Skin Types and Characteristics

Both the skin colour, which can vary from pale white to various shades of black, and the evenness of colour will affect and indicate sensitivity to external stimuli, ageing, UV radiation, hydration, facial hair growth and skin blemishes. Production of the skin pigment melanin varies across all skin types and characteristics. Black skins do not contain any more melanocytes than white skins do, but there are differences in the melanin granules in the differently coloured skins. In black skins the melanin granules are larger, where as in white skins they are less obvious

- ☐ **White skin** – fair in colour, often with freckles and accompanied by red, blonde or brown hair and green/blue eyes. Tends to be more sensitive to UV rays, and external stimuli, to age more quickly and show vascular disorder, for instance in a florid complexion. It is important to start to protect the skin from UV rays as early as possible.

- ☐ **Mixed skin** – a combination of some of the skin types; the shades and sensitivities will vary greatly depending upon the mix.

- ☐ **Asian-type skin** – predominantly yellow in tone with a sallow tinge. It is often oily but smooth and evenly coloured. Asian skin tends to age well but is more prone to hyperpigmentation from operation scars and lesions, so should be treated with care. This type of skin ages very well and does not line or wrinkle in the same way as white skin.

- ☐ **Black skin** – produce a large amount of melanin which determines the skin colour and depth of black skin. Although varying greatly in shades, black skin generally has greater protection from damaging UV rays, tends to be more supple with delayed ageing effects, but more reactive to stimuli such as rashes or inflammations which can leave dark marks and scarring on the skin. It is also more prone to keloid scarring. It is generally oily skin, but if it becomes dry, dead skin cells appear ashen.

- ☐ **Young skin** – looks even in colour, with fine, clear texture, soft, smooth and supple but firm, with a balance of oil and moisture. This skin type generally only needs protection and maintenance treatment.

- ☐ **Mature skin** – with age, the skin will lose firmness and elasticity, and may feel looser and thinner. This change in texture may cause the appearance of fine lines, and less definition of the contours of the face. The skin becomes dry, as the sebaceous glands become less active. As the skin appears thinner, becoming almost transparent in some areas such as around the eyes small capillaries can show through the skin. Waste products are removed less quickly than in a young skin, and this leads to puffiness of the skin particularly around the eyes. Patches of irregular pigmentation may appear on the surface of the skin such as lentigo and chloasma.

- ☐ **Oily skin** – may appear sallow and dull or shiny and hard (seborrhoea), with uneven texture and enlarged pores, particularly down the central T zone, with comedones (black heads) and papules. Due to an over-secretion of the sebaceous glands, often during adolescence and frequently affected by the menstrual cycle, it can occur at any time in areas of the face. Generally, treatments seek to unblock pores through specialised cleaning routines, but must avoid dehydrating the skin with harsh products.

- ☐ **Combination skin** – Can be a combination of any two skin types on the same face although there is generally a central oily zone, with the cheeks and neck showing normal or dry skin. This is a very common skin type, and there are products created specially for combination skin types.

- ☐ **Dry skin** – generally appears pale and thin, with fine lines, no visible pores, sometimes broken capillaries and flakiness. It may feel and look tight. It may be a result of dehydration, and, although more commonly associated with middle age, it can appear at any age and be caused by genetic, internal or external (such as sun tanning) factors. Treatments stimulate the dry skin to correct the oil and moisture balance.

Skin Conditions and Texture

Blemished skin tends to feel coarse and bumpy and may indicate present or previous skin conditions. Skin imperfections include:

- **dehydrated skin** – is skin that has lost water from the skin tissues. This condition can affect any skin type, the problem maybe related to the client's general health, lifestyle, diet and skin care regime. In many cases the dehydration can be caused by working environment with a low humidity, or in one that is air-conditioned. The skin has fine superficial lines, superficial flaking and broken capillaries are common.

- **sensitive skin** – can look like dry skin, usually with high colour and signs of dilated capillaries. It is easily stimulated, often becoming red and blotchy, and responds quickly to treatment, so care is needed. Treatments emphasise calming routines and products to maintain the skin's balance.

- **open pores** – due to oily skin or, in a mature client with dry skin, due to a previous skin condition.

- **broken capillaries (couperose)** – dilated capillaries on a fine skin texture often affecting large areas of the face indicating sensitive or thin skin. The skin responds fiercely to stimulation and permanent dilated vessels are apparent, particularly on the upper cheeks and nose. Ruptured blood vessels assume a line-like appearance in surface tissues and can become bulbous and blue in colour due to the congestion in the blood vessels of the area.

- **hyper pigmentation** – darker pigmented areas possibly indicating sun damage.

- **hypo pigmentation** – uneven patches of skin tone, lighter than the surrounding skin due to lack of melanin in the area.

- **dermatosis papulosa nigra** – also called flesh moles, these are brown or black hyper pigmentation markings resembling moles. The cause is unknown but sometimes found to be hereditary. It most frequently occurs on female black skin.

- **pseudo folliculitis** – an inflammatory skin disorder which mainly occurs in male black skins as the hair is coarser and curly and has a tendency as it grows out for the skin to curl back and re-enter the follicle becoming in growing making the skin irritated and inflamed. Hyper pigmentation may also accompany this condition.

- **keloids** – scarring that becomes enlarged and projects from the skin's surface, caused by hyperplasia.

- **scarring** – due to injury, chickenpox or post acne.

- **thin skin** – due, for instance, to steroid treatment for severe eczema.

- **small moles** – an abnormal collection of pigment cells present within the skin, melanocytes. Moles are extremely common and most people are born with a few and may develop others during their lives.

- **Birthmarks** – these marks can be red, pink, brown, tan or blue. There is no way to prevent birthmarks. They are not inherited and very little is known about how they occur.

- **lack of elasticity** – may be evident in lines that firstly appear around the eyes and maybe the mouth either naturally or prematurely. Oily skins are more likely to age better than a dry skin, although oily skins often suffer more with blemishes particularly during puberty.

- **lack of muscle tone** – dropped contours usually indicate a mature skin, as muscles become atrophied with age.

- **blemishes** – are marks on the skin, which may be temporary or permanent and may include any of the following, broken capillaries, comedones, milia, scarring, pigmentation spots and moles.

- **age** – refer to page 91 – *Ageing of the skin.*

- **crow's feet** – fine lines around the eyes caused by habitual expressions and daily movement, associated with ageing of muscle tissue. Premature formation may be due to eye strain and is often associated with oedema (swelling) around and under the eyes.

- **comedones** – commonly known as blackheads, these are caused by a build-up of sebaceous secretions which have become trapped in the hair follicles and have subsequently dried out and hardened. The colour comes from oxidation. Common in puberty.

- **milia** – commonly known as whiteheads, these form when sebum becomes trapped in a blind duct with no surface opening. The condition is most common on dry skin and milia appear on the obicularis oculi muscle area and between the eyebrows. Milia can form after injury, e.g. sunburn on the face or shoulders, and are sometimes widespread.

- **pustules** – a small inflamed elevation of the skin that is filled with fluid/pus.

- **papules** – a small, solid inflammatory elevation of the skin that does not contain pus.

- **ingrowing hairs** – when hairs begin to re-grow, particularly after waxing or shaving, they can curl up inside the hair follicle. The hair doubles over itself making it impossible for it to exit the surface. As the hair continues to grow inside the follicle it

creates a foreign body reaction. This causes inflammation and a red bump emerges on the surface of the skin.

Environmental and lifestyle factors that can affect the condition of the skin

- UV damage
- Diet
- Smoking
- Alcohol
- Central heating
- Air conditioning
- Stress
- Air travel
- Fresh air
- Sleep
- Exercise

KEY POINT

Skin imperfections are not necessarily contraindications to treatment, but therapists should advise the client to seek medical guidance if in any doubt about a blemish. Therapists must not offer a diagnosis.

Client consultation and initial visual check

See Chapter 1 for more detail on how to conduct professional and confidential client consultations. However, for skin treatments it is particularly important to obtain details on any contraindications, and helpful to understand aspects of your client's lifestyle that could be relevant to skin treatments. This information includes:

- lifestyle – a hectic or stressful lifestyle, unbalanced diet or too little sleep can affect the condition of the skin, for instance psoriasis may be associated with stress

- occupation – work environments which expose the skin to dust, wind, sun, central heating or air conditioning can all affect and damage skin

- health – poor general health, medication, and specific conditions such as eczema, can affect skin in a variety of ways

- skin-care routine – products, skin-care routines and any reactions to them that the client has noticed, can be important in deciding which products to use or the causes of a condition

- previous treatments – it is important to know about any previous treatments and any reactions to them

- your own initial visual check of the client's skin, which together with what the client tells you, should determine whether to proceed any further at this stage. If you do proceed, you will add to this with more detailed inspection

- what the client feels about their skin and if they know what treatment they would actually like.

This is also the time to set your client at ease, inform them about available and appropriate treatments, and give your professional advice; if necessary, refer your client on to medical advice.

Salon Name
Client Consultation Form – *Skincare and Eye Treatments*

Client Name: **Date:**

Address:

Profession:

e-mail: **Tel. No:** Day

                                                              Eve

---

PERSONAL DETAILS
Age group: Under 20☐ 20–30☐ 30–40☐ 40–50☐ 50–60☐ 60+☐
Lifestyle: Active ☐ Sedentary☐
Last visit to the doctor:
GP Address:
No. of children (if applicable):   **Date of last period (if applicable):**

CONTRAINDICATIONS REQUIRING MEDICAL PERMISSION – in circumstances where medical permission cannot be obtained clients must give their informed consent in writing prior to treatment. *(select if/where appropriate)*:

Medical oedema☐   Skin cancer☐
Nervous/Psychotic conditions☐   Slipped disc☐
Epilepsy☐   Undiagnosed pain☐
Recent operations affecting the area☐   Whiplash☐
Diabetes☐   When taking prescribed medication☐
Other:

CONTRAINDICTIONS THAT RESTRICT TREATMENT *(select if/where appropriate)*:

Fever☐   Scar tissue (2 years for major operation and 6 months for a small scar) ☐
Contagious or infectious diseases☐   Sunburn☐
Diarrhoea and vomiting☐   Hormonal implants☐
Under the influence of recreational drugs or alcohol☐   Recent fractures (minimum 3 months)☐
Skin allergies☐   Sinusitis☐
Eczema ☐   Neuralgia☐
Trapped/Pinched nerve affecting the treatment area☐   Any other condition affecting the neck☐
Inflamed nerve☐   Migraine/Headache☐
Undiagnosed lumps and bumps☐   Hypersensitive skin☐
Localised swelling☐   Broken capillaries☐
Inflammation☐   Botox/dermal fillers (1 week following treatment)☐
Cuts☐   Conjunctivitis☐
Bruises☐   Stye☐
Abrasions☐   Eye infection☐
                                             Watery eyes☐
                                             Hyper-keratosis☐
                                             Any known allergies☐

UNDERSTAND AND RECOGNISE OTHER CONDITIONS WHICH MAY AFFECT FACIAL TREATMENT *(select if/where appropriate)*:

Cardio vascular conditions (thrombosis, phlebitis, hypertension, heart conditions)☐   Bells Palsy☐
Any condition already being treated by a GP or another practitioner☐   Postural deformities☐
Arthritis☐   Acute rheumatism☐
Any dysfunction of the nervous system☐   Cervical spondylitis☐

CONTRAINDICTIONS FOR EYE TREATMENTS ONLY *(select if/where appropriate)*:

Any eye surgery (approx 6 months)☐   Watery eyes☐

Conjunctivitis☐   Blepharitis☐

Stye☐   Very nervous clients☐

Eye infection☐

Any previous reaction to eyelash/brow tint?   If yes, state type of reaction:

Reaction to patch test: Date of patch test: Product used:

SKIN TEST *(select if/where appropriate)*:

Moisture content:	Excellent☐	Good☐	Fair☐	Poor☐
Muscle tone:	Excellent☐	Good☐	Fair☐	Poor☐
Elasticity:	Excellent☐	Good☐	Fair☐	Poor☐
Sensitivity:	High☐	Medium☐	Low☐	
Skins healing ability:	Excellent☐	Good☐	Fair☐	Poor☐
Skin tone:	Fair☐	Medium☐	Dark☐	Olive☐
Circulation:	Good☐	Normal☐	Poor☐	
Pores:	Fine☐	Dilated☐	Comodones☐	Milia☐

Brief Description:

TREATMENT TO INCLUDE *(select if/where appropriate)*:

Superficial Cleanse☐ Deep Cleanse☐ Pre-Heat treatment☐ Skin Analysis☐

Lash Tinting☐ Brow Tinting☐ Eyebrow Tweezing☐ Massage☐ Mask☐

Therapist Signature...................................

Client Signature...

Clients Lifestyle:

Treatment details:

Home care advice:

Overall conclusion of the treatment:

Reflective practice:

Using the record card

See Chapter 1 for general use of the record card. In addition, for skin treatments:

☐ check for information about skin treatments and contraindications already on the record card

☐ re-analyse the skin type and condition before each skin treatment and note any findings and contraindications on the record card.

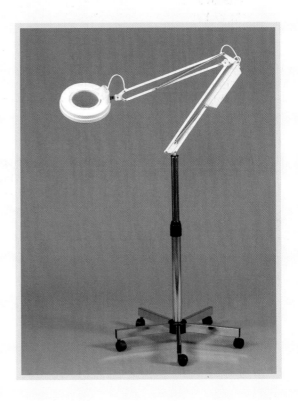

ENDPOINTS

You should now know:

☐ the methods for analysing skin type

☐ how to perform and record a client consultation and initial visual check.

Topic 3: Superficial cleansing treatments

Cleansing is the essential first step to any skin treatment. Following on from the initial observation, record card and communication with the client (see Topic 2), it will give the therapist detailed information of the client's skin condition and sensitivity. It can also be a soothing and relaxing treatment in its own right, and allow the client to become used to the feel of the therapist's touch.

> **KEY POINT**
> All observations of the skin, its reactions, the treatment and products used, should be recorded on the client's record card.

Using cleansing products

For effective cleansing that will not irritate the client's skin, the correct products must be used. The therapist must know the products' properties and effects, and should take into consideration:

☐ the client's skin type and condition (see Topic 2)

☐ the skin's sensitivity and allergic reactions (if known in advance)

☐ the products' texture and perfume, to be used according to the client's preference

☐ the products' effectiveness and appropriateness.

The main types of superficial cleansers available are lotions, milks and creams, many of which are based on natural ingredients.

Cleansing lotions – oil in water solutions that feel light, sharp and refreshing on the skin, and are recommended for oily and congested skins. Some can be removed with water.

Cleansing milks – oil-based emulsions with a high water content, making them flow easily on the skin. They can be formulated for all skin types, but are ideal for young/normal oily or combination skin types.

Cleansing creams – mainly water-in-oil emulsions, but with a much smaller water content than the milks, so are more oily and therefore more suitable for dry, mature skins or dehydrated skins.

Cleansing foams – for all skin types and usually very light in texture. Their foam or mousse consistency removes make-up quickly and avoids dragging mature skins. They can be washed off with water, leaving the skin feeling refreshed.

Cleansing gels – these alcohol-free gels lather well and have a strong degreasing action to remove excess oils without causing moisture loss. The gel is massaged over dry skin, then water is added to create a lather, before removing with a cloth, splashing and blotting dry.

> **KEY POINT**
> When using any product, always follow the manufacturer's instructions carefully.

Manual cleansing routine

1. Prepare your products and materials

Having decided which products you are going to use, make sure they are easily to hand. Then prepare damp cotton wool and tissues.

2. Prepare the client

Make sure the client's hair and clothing are protected, and that they are relaxed on the couch with eyes closed. Explain quietly what you will be doing and the products you will be using.

3. Eye make-up removal

Avoiding harsh or sudden movements, use the prepared damp cotton wool, soaked with eye make-up remover, to remove eye make-up quickly and efficiently by holding up the eyebrow gently but firmly with one hand, sweep gently downward and inwards with the other cotton wool pad. Turn the cotton wool at each stroke to use a clean surface, then lightly sweep under the lashes towards the nose. Repeat until all eye make-up has been thoroughly removed. Use separate pads for each eye to avoid cross-infection.

4. Lipstick removal

Fold a damp cotton wool pad. Holding one side of the mouth firmly in place, use the cotton wool pad to pass across the opposite side of the mouth with a light pressure, which does not pull or distort the mouth, to remove the lipstick. Reverse the procedure, using a clean cotton wool pad or turn it over, to remove the lipstick from the other side of the mouth.

5. Cleanser application

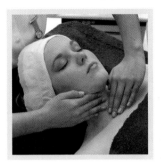 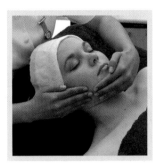
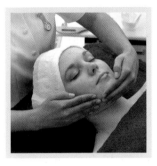 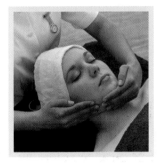

Select the appropriate cleanser for the client's skin type. Place a small amount in your hands and gently wipe it through your hands to spread it evenly and to warm it prior to application. Apply to the client's face in long sweeping effleurage stokes covering the whole of the face and neck.

Use superficial strokes to begin, altering the strokes for sensitive areas such as the upper cheeks, eyes and trachea (wind pipe), and for the forehead.

First mould the hands around the neck and decollete following the contours, gently moving up the neck to the jaw bone (mandible), then across the neck and decollete, returning and repeating more deeply.

In the chin area, concentrate first on one side then the other. Avoid distorting the mouth or touching the nose, but work the hands deeply into the chin fold.

Treat the nose next, with careful attention to removing all make-up in this area. Work into the creases using the finger tips. As you move across the upper cheekbones to the forehead, ease the pressure to lighter, calming movements.

Finish the routine with slow, gentle circles round the eyes and with gentle, even, upward pressure on the temples.

6. Cleanser removal

To remove cleanser use two damp cotton wool pads wrapped around the 3rd and 4th fingers, one in each hand. Start with the decollete, with your hands following each other or working one on each side. Then move to the cheeks, the nose and the forehead, turning and changing the pads as necessary, ending this part of the sequence with circles around the eyes and gentle pressure on the temples.

Always ensure cleansing movements are performed in an upward motion and never 'drag' the skin in any way.

Follow this with detailed removal from the central panel, with fresh pads wrapped around the 3rd and 4th fingers. Slowly and gently move up the forehead. Finally, open out the pads to the arches of the eyes.

Damp sponges, which can be sanitised and reused, can be used instead of disposable cotton wool pads for removal of cleanser. Meticulous sanitising methods must be used for sponges to avoid cross infections, and water must be changed regularly.

Repeat cleanse sequence.

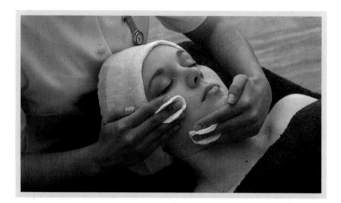

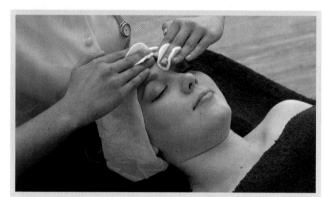

Toning the skin

Toning the skin is the second stage in most cleansing routines. As well as ensuring complete removal of cleansing preparations, toning is also used:

☐   to refine the skin

☐   to cool and refresh the skin

☐   to close the pores

☐   after a face mask, to remove all traces of the face mask

☐   before make-up, to allow a matt, long-lasting make-up to be applied.

Skin toning products

Skin fresheners – are the mildest of the toning products, they usually contain little or no alcohol, and mainly consist of purified water with floral extract such as rose water or chamomile. Recommended for dry, delicate, sensitive and mature skins.

Skin tonics – are slightly stronger than the skin fresheners, may contain an astringent agent such as witch hazel. Recommended for normal and combination skins.

Astringents – are the strongest of all the toners, and have a high proportion of alcohol. They may contain antiseptic ingredients such as hexachlorophene, which is particularly beneficial to promote healing for a blemished skin. Recommended for oily, blemished and acne skins with no sensitivity.

☐ Some astringents contain antiseptic substances to kill bacteria, dry and heal pustules and prevent blackheads forming.

☐ Astringents containing alcohol are the strongest toners; they irritate the skin causing it to swell around the pores so that they look temporarily less obvious.

☐ Astringents are too strong for dry, sensitive, mature skins as they dry out the skin's surface.

Manual skin toning

When you have matched the toner to both the cleanser and the client's skin type, gently apply toner, avoiding sensitive areas if necessary.

Toner can be applied using:

☐ dampened cotton wool pads and an opened-out tissue to dry the skin.

☐ a gauze toning compress soaked in lotion and applied to the skin for a few minutes

☐ an aerosol spray, using skin fresheners mixed with distilled water, sprayed in a fine mist over the face and neck. Use a paper tissue placed over the face, held gently against the skin, to absorb excess moisture.

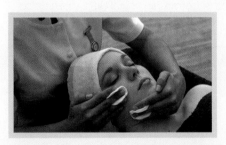

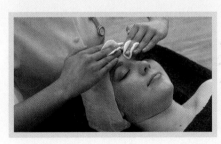

ENDPOINTS
You should now know how to:

☐ use cleansing products

☐ tone the skin.

Topic 4: Pre-heat treatments

It is a good idea to warm and soften the skin with hot towels or a facial steamer. These make it easier to remove comedones (blackheads) and excess sebum from the pores. Steaming can be used as either a pre-heat treatment or a precursor to a deep-cleanse treatment.

Using hot towels

Fold a towel in half and half again, then soak one end of the folded towel in hot water. Always ensure the temperature is appropriate for the client's skin.

Roll up the towel from the wet end, then squeeze it out. Open the towel out and fold it carefully around your client's face leaving the nostrils free to breathe. Press it gently to mould it to the face.

Using hot towels from a hot-towel cabinet may be preferred to steaming as a pre-heat treatment. Pressure points may be used whilst the towel is on the client's face, and this can also be very relaxing for clients who do not mind having their eyes covered.

Removing comedones and milia

The best time to remove comedones or milia is when the skin has been softened with hot towels or steaming.

Remove comedones with your fingers, covered in tissues or cotton wool.

1. With your fingers cleaned and covered with soft facial tissue or cotton wool gently roll and squeeze the area around the blockage until it comes out of the follicle, without breaking the skin.

2. Wipe away the waste with a clean tissue and wipe over the open pores with a mild antiseptic to avoid infection.

Milia appear as small, white pearly nodules on the skin.

1. Do not attempt to squeeze out milia.

2. Milia should not be lanced, use massage, exfoliation and steaming to soften the blockage and open the pore.

3. Take great care to minimise skin damage and prevent infection.

4. Remove waste with a clean tissue, then wipe over with a mild antiseptic.

Do not attempt to lance or squeeze cysts. These appear as swellings under the skin. Advise a client with a large cyst to seek medical advice.

ENDPOINTS
You should now know how to:

☐ use hot towels

☐ remove comedones and milia.

Topic 5: Deep-cleansing skin treatments

Deep-cleansing treatments are generally seen as essential preparations for further treatments, but they can also be beneficial and relaxing or stimulating treatments in their own right.

Deep cleansing takes place after the initial cleansing and skin analysis have revealed your client's individual skin type. You can then choose a suitable technique or programme and products for deep cleansing the skin. Deep cleansing methods include:

☐ steaming

☐ brush cleaning

☐ using AHAs

☐ exfoliation creams

We will look at masks in Topic 11.

Steaming (without ozone)

Steaming is beneficial to all skin types and can form part of any cleansing routine.

Contraindications for steaming

See Chapter 1 for general contraindications. Contraindications specific to steaming are:

☐ skin infections

☐ sunburn

☐ acne rosacea

☐ extreme vascularity (broken capillaries) or hypersensitive skin

☐ sinus blockage

☐ Claustrophobia.

General effects and benefits of steaming

Steaming has many general cleansing benefits, it:

☐ opens the pores and softens the skin, preparing it for further treatment

☐ stimulates sudoriferous glands to produce sweat, eliminating waste

☐ softens the oily deposits in follicles making it easier to remove comedones

☐ increases circulation and temperature, improving skin colour

☐ softens dead skin cells, aiding desquamation (removal of dead cells)

☐ prepares skin for further treatment.

Uses and benefits according to client's skin type

In addition to the general benefits, steaming is used for particular effects for the different skin types. Skin type will also determine the distance of the steamer head from the client and the length of time the steamer is used.

For young skin – use for 5–10 minutes to maintain skin texture.

For dry or mature skin – use for about 5 minutes to hydrate, desquamate, regenerate cells and improve skin colour.

For sensitive skin – use for about 3–5 minutes to hydrate and gently cleanse.

For oily skin – use for about 10 minutes to unblock congestion, deep cleanse and improve skin colour.

Do not use on sensitive skin

Using the steamer

1. Preparing the equipment

☐ Check the water level.

☐ If necessary, fill the water reservoir with distilled water (tap water would allow deposits to build up).

☐ Switch the steamer on 10 minutes before it is needed facing away from the client and therapist allowing the water to heat up – you can use this time for superficial cleansing and preparing your client.

☐ When it starts to steam, switch off the steamer until you are ready to use it.

2. Preparing your client

☐ Place your client in a semi-reclining position. Your client should not be lying flat for a steam treatment.

☐ Cover the hair to protect it from moisture.

☐ Protect your client's eyes, sensitive skin areas and any areas of high colour with cotton wool pads.

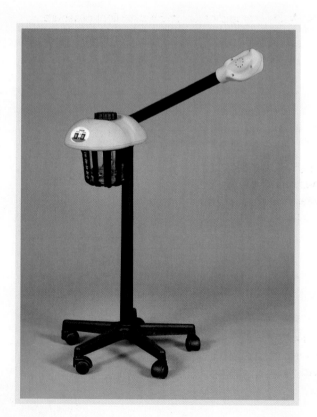

3. Using the steamer

☐ Switch the steamer back on and position its head appropriately to allow the steam to flow over the client's face and neck. This should be a maximum of 18 inches from the highest point (nose).

☐ Adjust the steamer as necessary to cover different areas.

☐ Do not keep the steamer on longer than the recommended times for the different skin types (see above and refer to the manufacturer's instructions).

☐ Watch the skin for any reactions and shorten the time if necessary.

☐ When the required treatment is finished, switch off the steamer and move its head away from your client before removing the eye pads.

☐ Blot off the surface skin moisture.

KEY POINT

As with most treatments, always keep a careful eye on your client's progress and reactions and adjust timing accordingly. Never leave a client on their own.

Steaming with ozone

Most facial steamers can produce steam on their own or combined with ozone.

Ozone is produced when the oxygen in the steam is passed over a high-intensity quartz mercury arc tube. The effects of steaming with ozone are:

☐ Drying

☐ Antibacterial/germicidal

☐ Promotes healing

☐ Helps to normalise the Ph of the skin

Ozone steaming is beneficial for oily, blemished or congested skins, but should be used with caution, as it is thought to be carcinogenic. Always follow manufacturer's instructions and use in a well-ventilated room for a minimum amount of time.

Brush cleansing

Electrical brush cleansing is a popular deep-cleansing routine because it is quick and benefits all but the most sensitive skin types. It is usually used after a manual or steam cleanse.

Contraindications

See Topic 1 for more information on general contraindications. Those specifically for electrical brush cleansing are:

☐ acne vulgaris

☐ acne rosacea

☐ sensitive skin with broken capillaries

☐ bruising, cuts and abrasions

☐ new scar tissue.

Benefits of brush cleansing

Brush cleansing is beneficial because it:

☐ gently removes dead surface skin cells

☐ removes cellular blockages

☐ improves skin colour

☐ improves cellular regeneration.

Preparing your client

Usually your client will have had a manual and/ or steam cleanse before the brush cleanse to remove make-up. Your client will lie on the couch during the treatment.

☐ Make sure your client's hair is fully covered so it cannot catch in the brushes and will not be affected by the cleansing preparation.

☐ Ask your client to close her eyes and cover the eyes with damp cotton wool pads to prevent cleansing preparation from going in them.

☐ With a circular mask brush, generously apply a cleansing medium, such as a water-based cleansing milk or a medium appropriate to your client's skin type:

– for oily/blemished skin use cleansing foam

– for oily/combination skin use a cleansing lotion

– for dry/mature/sensitive skin use a cleansing cream.

Using the brushes

Brush-cleansing units vary from small hand-held units to individual or combined machines. There are a variety of brushes to suit different skin types, and the speed and direction of brush rotation can be varied.

☐ Always soften the brushes with water before use.

☐ Choose an appropriate size brush head for skin area, e.g.:

– a larger brush head for the neck

– a small brush head for sides of the nose.

☐ Choose soft, tapered brushes for cleansing and for dry/sensitive skin.

☐ Choose firm, bristly brushes for activating and abrasive massage.

When switched on, the chosen applicator (brush) gently vibrates and rotates.

☐ Apply the applicator gently, with light pressure, following the contours of the face.

☐ Use the minimum number of strokes.

☐ Reduce the pressure and speed over bony areas.

☐ Use slower speeds on dry/sensitive skin.

☐ Use faster speeds on coarser skin with a thick epidermis.

When the procedure is finished, remove the cleansing medium with damp cotton wool pads (see Topic 3 Cleanser removal). You can now continue with the facial routine or apply moisturiser.

KEY POINT

After use, clean the brushes thoroughly in hot, soapy water; disinfect them and store them in a dry sanitiser, eg UV or chemical.

Using AHA cleansers (fruit acid peels)

AHAs (alpha hydroxy acids) are mild, organic, natural acids found in citrus fruit, bilberries, sugar and milk. They are used in creams, cleansers and moisturisers for a range of skin restorative effects. AHAs had been used for centuries to reverse the ageing process before their effectiveness was recognized by modern science.

☐ AHAs help to loosen dead skin cells on the skin's surface, which:

- – increases speed of removal of dead cells (desquamation)
- – increases speed of renewal of cells
- – improves texture and condition of skin

☐ AHAs increase the skin's natural moisture-holding ability

☐ AHAs improve the appearance of fine lines and wrinkles.

Alpha hydroxy acids are familiar to all of us:

☐ Lactic acid is found in milk

☐ Oranges and lemons contain citric acid

☐ Apples – malic acid

☐ Aged wine is rich in tartaric acid

☐ Glycolic acid is extracted from sugar cane

AHAs are natural, not only are they found in plants and natural foods, but also in the human body. However the quantity of AHAs produced by our bodies is not sufficient to combat wrinkles.

Did you know?

Cleopatra used to bathe in asses' milk, believing that it would keep her skin soft and fresh.

Used as deep-cleansing lotions or masks, AHAs are particularly recommended for dry, mature skin, oily or open pores, and dehydration.

Safety note

When first introduced, high concentration AHAs caused some cases of high erythema irritation and skin damage.

Concentrations of less than 10% fruit acids and pH higher than 3.5 are now used quite safely. However, some clients may feel a mild tingling or itching during treatment and have a mild erythema for a short time afterwards. Explain to them that this is quite normal. If a client feels stronger discomfort, remove the AHA swiftly.

Exfoliation creams

Exfoliation creams are facial scrubs with fine exfoliating particles, such as oatmeal, crushed nut kernels and pumice, to soften and remove the dead skin cells and any impurities. They combine a detergent cleansing action with gentle abrasion.

Using exfoliation creams

1. Dampen the skin if recommended by the product supplier.

2. Apply with the fingertips.

3. Massage over the skin to loosen dead cells and other surface impurities. Use small, circular movements, starting on the décolleté, then the face and ending on the forehead.

4. Rinse off the skin with clean, warm water.

Benefits of exfoliation creams

Exfoliation creams:

☐ brighten the complexion and refine the skin texture

☐ help reverse some of the damage of too much sun by evening out the coarse surface

☐ help combat dryness and premature wrinkles

☐ stimulate the blood supply

☐ leave the skin soft, smooth and clean.

All skin types can benefit from different types of exfoliation creams.

Record card

Carefully record all treatments, including:

☐ products and procedures used

☐ any contraindications and reactions to treatment

☐ advice for after care given.

☐ home care advice given and any products sold.

ENDPOINTS

You should now know the procedures for:

☐ steaming

☐ brush cleansing

☐ using AHA cleansers

☐ using exfoliation creams

Topic 6: Eyebrow shaping

Eyebrows frame the eyes and show them off to their best advantage when pleasingly shaped. Depending on the needs of the individual client, eyebrow shaping and eyebrow and/or eyelash tinting can be offered either as individual stand-alone treatments, or they can be incorporated into a full facial treatment.

Contraindications

Before you begin this treatment, check for the following contraindications.

Contraindications requiring medical permission – in circumstances where medical permission cannot be obtained clients must give their informed consent in writing prior to the treatment

- ☐ Medical oedema
- ☐ Nervous/Psychotic conditions
- ☐ Epilepsy
- ☐ Recent facial operations affecting the area
- ☐ Diabetes
- ☐ Skin cancer
- ☐ Slipped disc
- ☐ Undiagnosed pain
- ☐ When taking prescribed medication
- ☐ Whiplash

Contraindications that restrict treatment

- ☐ Fever
- ☐ Contagious or infectious diseases
- ☐ Under the influence of recreational drugs or alcohol
- ☐ Diarrhoea and vomiting
- ☐ Any known allergies
- ☐ Eczema
- ☐ Undiagnosed lumps and bumps
- ☐ Localised swelling
- ☐ Inflammation
- ☐ Cuts, bruises, abrasions
- ☐ Scar tissues (2 years for major operation and 6 months for a small scar)
- ☐ Hormonal implants
- ☐ Recent fractures (minimum 3 months)
- ☐ Sinusitis
- ☐ Neuralgia
- ☐ Sunburn
- ☐ Migraine/Headache
- ☐ Hypersensitive skin
- ☐ Botox/dermal fillers (1 week following treatment)
- ☐ Hyper-keratosis
- ☐ Skin allergies
- ☐ Styes
- ☐ Watery eyes
- ☐ Trapped/pinched nerve affecting the treatment area
- ☐ Inflamed nerve
- ☐ Eye infection
- ☐ Conjunctivitis
- ☐ Blepharitis

It is important to be aware of the appearance and cause of the main contraindications which relate specifically to eyes:

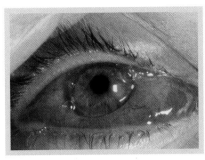

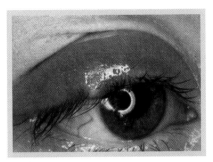

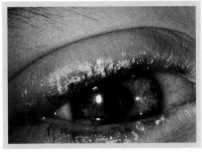

Conjunctivitis

The eyes will be red, sore and itching. This eye condition is usually caused by bacteria, but can be due to a virus or an allergy.

Stye

There will be a small, raised boil at the base of an eyelash follicle, and the eye will appear red, sore and swollen.

Blepharitis

The eye will look red and sore, due to infection of the eyelid

Viral infection

The client will have all the symptoms of a common cold or 'flu – sneezing, blocked nose, runny eyes etc.

Bruising

Bruising on and around the eye area can show as a variety of colours, including black, blue, purple and yellow.

Fresh scar tissue around eye area

If there is fresh scar tissue around the eye area, do not treat. Generally, scar tissue (on any area of the body) should be at least six months old for a small scar and two years for a large one before a treatment is performed in that area.

Reasons for eyebrow shaping

The main reasons why clients choose to have their eyebrows shaped are that the treatment will:

- ☐ tidy and define the brow line by producing a clean eyebrow shape

- ☐ accentuate the eyes

- ☐ ensure that eye make-up – especially eye shadow – can be used to better effect.

A face without groomed eyebrows has an unfinished, incomplete look.

Choosing the appropriate eyebrow shape

Before you start shaping the eyebrow, you will need to consider:

- ☐ the correct eyebrow width for the client
- ☐ the shape of the client's face and eyes
- ☐ the age of the client
- ☐ the client's own preference.

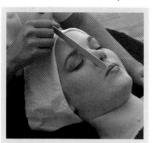 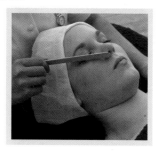

1. Determining the correct eyebrow width

You can determine the correct width for the client's eyebrows by using an orange wood stick to measure where the eyebrow should start and finish:

a. Place an orange wood stick in a straight line from the side of the nose to the inner corner of the eye. The eyebrow should not extend beyond this line. Tweeze any stray hairs out.

b. Place an orange wood stick to make a vertical line through the centre of the pupil when the client is looking straight ahead. This should form the natural high point of the arch of the eyebrow.

c. Place an orangewood stick so that it makes a diagonal line from the nose across to the outer corner of the client's eye. The eyebrow should not extend beyond this point. Tweeze any stray hairs out.

The way to measure is illustrated below.

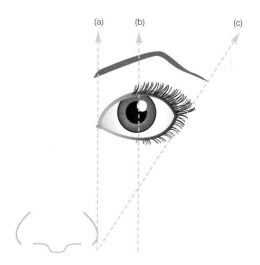

2. Determining the correct eyebrow shape to suit the client's eye shape and face shape

Eyebrows can be:

 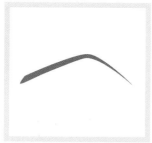 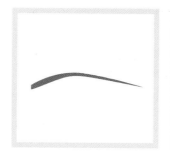 

1. Round/naturally shaped Face and eye shapes

2. An arched shape Face and eye shapes

3. Straight Face and eye shapes

4. Angular Face and eye shapes

1. Determining the correct eyebrow shape to suit the client's age

For older clients, be aware that heavy, thick eyebrows can be ageing, whilst thin eyebrows can give a very severe appearance to the face.

2. Determining the client's own preference

It is vital that, as with any other service provided to a client, you carefully consult with them so that, together, you can decide on the final eyebrow shape in accordance with their preferences, but also taking into account the natural shape of the brow.

There are two different kinds of tweezers that are used for eyebrow shaping:

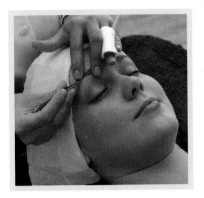 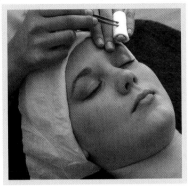 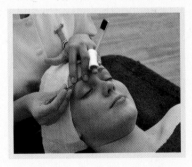

1. Manual tweezers

These are used to remove the bulk of the hairs and for fine work when defining the eyebrow shape.

2. Automatic tweezers

These are not often used in the salon. They have a spring-loaded action and are used to remove the bulk of excess hair.

Preparing the client for eyebrow shaping

The steps that should follow when preparing a client for an eyebrow shaping treatment are:

1. Check for contraindications.

2. Consult with the client to determine what they want to achieve.

3. Agree with the client the final eyebrow shape and appearance.

4. Secure the client's hair out of the way, using a headband or turban.

5. Ask the client to remove earrings, hair combs and pins, spectacles, or contact lenses (if worn).

6. Protect the client with towels or a cape, making sure that their clothes are completely covered.

7. Seat the client comfortably on a couch or chair.

8. Check that the client is at ease and ready for the treatment to begin.

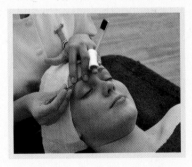

The tweezers you intend to use **must** be sterilised before the treatment commences. Sterilisation may have been carried out in the autoclave, bead steriliser or by soaking in a sterilising solution. If you do not use sterilised tweezers you run the risk of cross infection. Gloves should always be worn when performing this treatment.

Eyebrow shaping – carrying out the treatment

1. Use a suitable cleanser to remove all traces of face and eye make-up. Wipe over with sanitiser.

2. Use an orange stick to determine the appropriate width of the eyebrows.

3. Check with the client that you both understand and agree the shaping work that is to be carried out.

4. Give the client a hand mirror so that they can check progress whenever they choose.

5. Make sure that you always wear gloves when carrying out this treatment.

THE ART AND SCIENCE OF BEAUTY THERAPY

6. Apply cotton wool pads that have been soaked in warm water to the eyebrow area. The damp heat of the cotton wool will help to relax the hair follicles and soften the eye tissue. This will make it easier to remove the hairs; it will also make the process less painful and more comfortable for the client. Alternatively, when incorporating an eyebrow shape within a full facial treatment, it would be more comfortable for the client if you perform the tweeze immediately after facial steaming as this will be when the pores are open.

7. Begin by working on the stray hairs that grow on the bridge of the nose, between the client's eyes.

8. To tweeze, gently stretch the skin using your index and middle fingers, and with the tweezers remove hairs in the direction in which they are growing. NEVER remove hairs from above the brow. You will lose the natural pathway of the brow.

9. As you work, place the removed hairs onto a clean tissue or sterile cotton wool pad wrapped around the ring finger of the opposite hand.

10. Pause from time to time to allow your client to check progress in the hand mirror and to brush the hairs into place to check the progress of the brow shape.

11. As you work, wipe the client's brow with the cotton wool pad soaked in sanitiser. This will also help to remove any stray hairs that have fallen from the tweezers.

12. When both you and the client are completely satisfied with the finished shape, wipe the area you have been working on with a damp cotton wool pad which has been soaked in distilled water to calm and soothe the area.

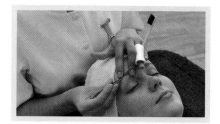 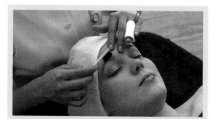 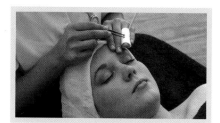

KEY POINT
Make sure that the tweezers and any other equipment used during this treatment are immediately sent for sterilisation so they cannot be used for another client.

Aftercare advice for your client
Following an eyebrow shaping treatment, advise your client that:

☐ they should not apply make-up to the treated area for at least twelve hours. This is because the pores will remain open for some time and infection from cosmetics could occur if they get into the open pores

☐ they can use distilled water to cool and soothe the area, if they choose.

Record keeping
Keeping accurate records of dates, procedures and products, including any contra-action that may have arisen during treatment, on the client's record card, is essential for consistency of practice and safety.

ENDPOINTS
You should now understand:

☐ the contraindications to eyebrow shaping

☐ the reasons why a client might choose to have their eyebrows shaped

☐ how to select the appropriate eyebrow shape for the client

☐ how to prepare the client for eyebrow shaping

☐ how to carry out an eyebrow shaping treatment

☐ what aftercare advice to give your client

☐ the importance of keeping appropriate records.

Topic 7: Eyebrow and eyelash tinting

Often combined as a treatment with eyebrow shaping and before facial massage, eyebrow and eyelash tinting is used to enhance the appearance through defining and correcting brow shapes, and emphasising lashes with colour.

Contraindications

Please see the contraindications for eyebrow shaping in Topic 6.

In addition, be aware of the following contraindications:

☐ tinting must always take place before eyebrow shaping to avoid any tint dropping into the open pores of the eyebrows and causing infection

☐ allergic reaction to patch test for tinting: as chemicals are used for tinting, a patch test MUST be performed approximately 48 hours before treatment using the same product line as is to be used for the treatment.

The patch test

The patch test should ideally take place 48 hours before treatment, and no longer than a week, as changes in the body can make the skin sensitive to products at different times. Skin may even become sensitive to particular products over time, during pregnancy or if medication is being taken.

1 Performing the patch test

☐ Mix a small quantity of the darkest tint and the appropriate percentage of hydrogen peroxide to be used.

☐ Apply with a brush or cotton bud to a small area of skin either behind the ear or in the crease of the elbow.

☐ After 48 hours, if no irritation has occurred (a negative reaction), wash off the tint.

☐ If redness, irritation or swelling occurs (a positive reaction), wash off the tint – which should stop the irritation – and apply a damp compress or suitable aftercare lotion.

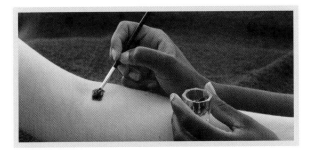

2 Producing written evidence of the patch test

☐ Include the following details on the client's record card:

☐ date and time of the patch test

☐ chemicals and dilutions used

☐ tint colour

☐ the appearance of the skin after the tint has been applied, including any contraindications, such as swelling, redness, irritation

☐ details of any treatment used to alleviate irritation, if it has occurred.

> **KEY POINT**
> If the client develops any kind of allergic reaction to the patch test – redness, swelling, itching – do not proceed with the treatment.

Reasons for choosing eyebrow and eyelash tinting

Tinting is often an alternative to mascara for:

☐ clients who are sensitive to eye make-up

☐ contact lens wearers whose eyes are irritated by fibres in mascara

☐ clients whose sporting activities, such as swimming, make mascara impractical

☐ clients who don't have time to apply eye make-up.

Tinting is also used:

☐ to increase colour intensity, especially for clients with blonde, red or grey hair or when clients are going on holiday.

☐ to give definition to fine or thin eyebrows.

Assessing the client's colouring

It is important to choose the appropriate colour and intensity of the tint. Blue, grey, brown and black colours in different applications can produce many shades and colour tones to suit the client's characteristics, hair and skin colouring.

☐ For mature and fair-skinned clients, softer colours produce a more natural look.

☐ Black is too harsh on blondes or redheads so grey or brown would be preferable.

☐ On dark-haired clients, blue tint added to black can add shine and a deeper colour.

☐ The base colour of the hairs affects the density of the final colour.

☐ A natural shade will help define dark brows at the outer corners, or blend in white hairs, to give a uniform tone and more distinct profile to the brow.

☐ Lashes are usually tinted a darker tone than brows. Dark lashes will look longer with a dark tint on the lighter ends.

☐ As well as hair colour, take into consideration the client's skin tone – fair, medium, dark or olive – when choosing the appropriate tint.

☐ Always consult closely with the client about their preferences for colour and tone while giving advice about the final effect.

Preparing the client for eyebrow and eyelash tinting

In addition:

☐ consult with the client about the result they would like to achieve, and agree colours and areas to be tinted

☐ apply a film of petroleum jelly under the bottom lashes and around the eyebrows

☐ position manufactured pre-shaped shields or damp cotton pads shaped to the eye under the bottom lashes

☐ advise the client not to open their eyes once the protective layers are in place.

☐ apply protective film on the eyelid close to the lashes.

Mixing the tint

The tint colour is mixed with 10% hydrogen peroxide.

- Always check and follow the manufacturer's instructions for mixing the tint. On average one centimetre of tint and two drops of hydrogen peroxide is sufficient for brow and lash tinting; with experience and following the manufacturer's instructions, mixing the right amount of tint will minimise product wastage.

- Apply the tint immediately after mixing or the tinting will not be effective.

- The mixed tint should form an even-coloured, smooth emulsion.

Carrying out the treatment – eyelash and eyebrow tinting

When they are done together, eyelash tinting is normally applied before eyebrow tinting.

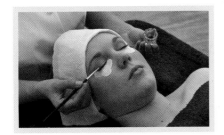 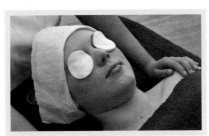 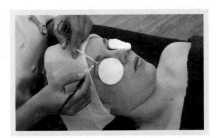

- Ensure the client's eyes remain closed until the end of the treatment.

- Check that the damp cotton wool pads or shields are neatly in place beneath the lower lashes, and apply more petroleum jelly to the eyelid if necessary.

- Apply eyelash tint with a tipped orange wood stick, tint brush or cotton bud.

- Carefully ensure the tint covers the roots as well as the ends of the lashes. It only needs to coat the lashes; anything more will not be absorbed and is wasted. The more tint that is applied, the more there is to remove, so avoid wastage.

- Apply dry cotton wool eye pads.

- Allow up to ten minutes development time or in accordance with manufacturer's instructions for the lashes, depending on the natural tone and the finish required.

- Remove the tint thoroughly with damp cotton wool and either tipped orange wood sticks or damp

cotton buds, using downward strokes onto the protective pad until the lashes are clean and no visible tint remains.

- Make a final check on the roots of the lashes with the client's eyes open. If there is still tint remaining, support the skin with one hand while removing the tint gently with a cotton wool tip.

Brow tinting is so quick it can be on and off whilst the lashes are still taking.

- Prepare the eyebrow area by applying a barrier cream around the eyebrow area to protect the skin

- Use a tipped orange wood stick, tint brush or cotton bud to apply the tint.

- Apply the tint first to the underneath brow hairs to ensure complete coverage. This can be achieved by first back brushing the eyebrow hairs and holding them up with an orange wood stick. Paint underneath the hairs then release them and paint the top of the hairs. This should be completed in sections working along the eyebrows.

115

☐ When the first brow is complete, start immediately on the second brow.

☐ Keep a visual check on the coloration of the first brow.

☐ Immediately the second brow is finished, remove the tint from the first brow with a damp cotton wool pad using firm wiping strokes.

☐ Ensure that no tint remains on the brow.

☐ Repeat the removal procedure for the second brow.

☐ Remember that red and white hair may require more time.

Contra-actions during treatment

Sometimes, even with a negative patch test, a client may experience an allergic reaction during treatment.

☐ If any contra-action occurs, stop treatment immediately and wipe off the tint with damp cotton pads.

☐ Any tint that touches the skin must be removed promptly to avoid skin staining, even through the protective petroleum jelly.

☐ An eyewash should only be used by a qualified first-aider.

Aftercare for the client

Tints last about six to eight weeks depending on hair growth. If repeating the procedure after this time, the client's skin may have changed in its sensitivity to the products and repeated patch tests are necessary at regular intervals, or if the client is pregnant or on medication.

Record keeping

Keeping accurate records on the client's record card of dates, procedures and products, including any contra-action that may have arisen during treatment, is essential for consistency of practice and safety.

See Chapter 1 for why this is especially important for eye treatments.

ENDPOINTS
You should now understand:

☐ the contraindications to eyelash or eyebrow tinting

☐ how to perform, assess, and record the results of a patch test

☐ the reasons why a client might choose to have their eyelashes or eyebrows tinted

☐ how to select the appropriate eyebrow shape for the client

☐ how to assess the client's colouring

☐ how to prepare the client for eyelash or eyebrow tinting

☐ how to mix the tint

☐ how to carry out an eyelash or eyebrow tinting treatment

☐ what contra-actions to look for during treatment

☐ what aftercare advice to give your client

☐ the importance of keeping appropriate records.

Topic 8:
The massage medium

Massage is usually thought to be the most relaxing treatment. It can benefit all clients and can be combined with many other treatments. Regular facial massage helps reduce the effects of stress, tension and tiredness, and desquamates, revitalises and tones facial contours. The main mediums for massage are:

☐ oils.

☐ creams.

There are many different types of oil and cream and it is important to choose a massage medium that is appropriate to your client's skin type and condition (see Topic 3). In addition, in order to work effectively, the medium should be:

☐ light

☐ non-sticky

☐ easily absorbed, but not so that it has become dry before the end of the massage

☐ not too runny

☐ a pleasant odour, or odourless.

Oils

Oils provide a good 'slip' for massage, stopping your fingers from dragging or stretching the skin. The most commonly used oils are:

☐ grape seed

☐ apricot kernel

☐ almond.

Safety

Check that your client does not have a nut allergy before using any nut-based products, such as almond oil.

Oils are especially appropriate for dry, sensitive and mature skins. To be effective, oils should:

☐ penetrate the skin easily

Examples of some oils and their benefits include:

☐ aloe vera, jojoba, evening primrose oil – for eczema and psoriasis

☐ calendula – for healing irritated skin

☐ almond, avocado – for dry, dehydrated skins.

Creams

Massage creams can contain many different ingredients and be of different textures for specific effects depending on your client's skin type and condition (see Topic 3).

For dry/mature skins – a rich cream to nourish the skin with a light enough consistency to prevent dragging the skin.

For sensitive skins – specially formulated massage creams that will not aggravate the skin and soothe any high colour or broken capillaries

For young skins – most mediums, not too heavy

For oily skins – creams with a higher water to oil ratio

Record card

Remember always to note in your client's record card:

☐ the massage medium you have used

☐ your client's response to it (for instance, liking/ disliking the perfume or texture)

☐ any skin reactions.

ENDPOINTS

At the end of this topic you should understand:

☐ the uses of oils as a massage medium

☐ the uses of creams as a massage medium

☐ the key points of record-keeping in massage.

Topic 9: Classical massage movements

In this topic we shall go through the different classical massage movements looking at techniques for applying them, when they should be used in the massage sequence, and their benefits.

One of our most instinctive reactions to a bump or blow is to rub the affected area. This basic human response has been developed into the techniques and procedures of modern massage.

The history of massage dates back for centuries. The earliest records of practice are from the ancient Chinese in 3000BC, and there is a steady stream of references through the centuries in Japanese, Indian, Greek, Roman, and renaissance European literature.

The ancient Chinese called their technique 'amma' and used specific movements at specific points on the body. The Japanese used a similar system, called 'tsubo' from which is descended modern Shiatsu massage.

For the Greeks and the Romans, massage was an integral part of an everyday regime of exercise and fitness. At Roman baths (as in Turkish baths today) massage was an important part of the ritual.

The beginnings of modern massage can be said to date from 1813, when Per Henrik Ling established the Royal Central Institute of Gymnastics in Sweden, formalising the sequences of movements and techniques, including 'effleurage' or stroking, 'petrisage' or pressing and squeezing and 'tapotement' or tapping, which we know as Swedish massage. Through the nineteenth and early twentieth centuries the therapeutic practise of massage battled against image and public perception, until the efforts of the Society of Trained Masseuses and later the Chartered Institute of Physiotherapy lead to a resurgence in it's use in rehabilitation and the treatment of nerve injuries.

Massage is now a respectable and respected therapy, based on many systems, but the principles of Swedish massage remain at the heart of most therapeutic practice.

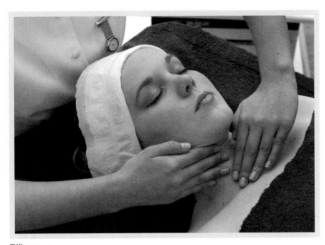

Effleurage

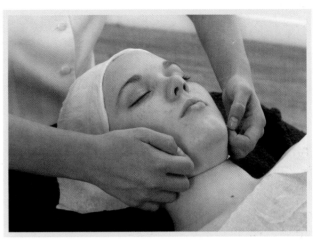

Petrissage (kneading)

Effleurage

Stroking movements

Pressure – light or firm, without dragging skin; gentle, even, surface pressure

When – beginning (to distribute cream or oil), end, and linking between movements

Using – palm surface and pads of fingers (not tips); hand relaxed

Effects of light effleurage:

- ☐ spreads the medium and introduces the client to the therapists touch
- ☐ improves skin texture
- ☐ is less relaxing than deep effleurage

Effects of deep effleurage:

- ☐ increases circulation
- ☐ nourishes skin
- ☐ removes waste/aids desquamation
- ☐ increases lymph flow
- ☐ soothes and relaxes, in particular the muscular and nervous system.

Petrissage

Movements – Palmar kneading, thumb kneading, finger kneading, knuckling, rolling, pinching (pincement)

Pressure – deeper pressure generally; lighter pressure over bony areas

When – after initial effleurage, and throughout massage, concentrating on different muscles particulary good for tension in the neck and shoulders

Using – pads of the fingers and/or thumbs; whole palm or surface of the hands

Effects of petrissage:

- ☑ increases circulation
- ☑ aids desquamation
- ☑ improves skin texture
- ☐ improves muscle tone (deeper pressure)
- ☐ relaxes muscles – releasing muscular tension
- ☑ stimulates circulation

Petrissage includes many different movements which, with practice, you will be able to perfect and adapt to suit your individual clients.

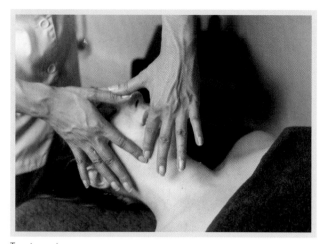

Tapotement

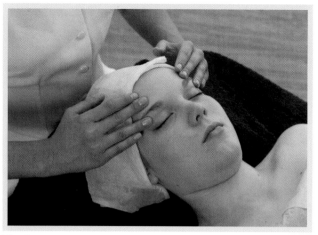

Vibrations

Tapotement – percussion

Tapotement produces a stimulating action on the tissues.

Movements – quick, even tapping

Pressure– light, quick

When –Towards the end of the treatment in particular areas which require toning , such as under the mandible and around the eyes

Using – pads of two fingers together – tapping

Ulna border of the hands alternately – hacking

Pincement – pinching along the cheeks and mandible

Effects of tapotement:

- ☐ increases blood supply to specific areas
- ☐ increases muscle tone
- ☐ reduces nervous tension
- ☐ stimulates nerve endings, revitalising tissue

Safety: do not use tapotement over dilated capillaries.

Vibrations

Movements – fine trembling caused by rapidly contracting and relaxing your hand and arm muscles producing light vibrations; either over one place or travelling over an area

Pressure – light

When – towards the end of the massage

Using – fingertips

Effects of vibrations:

- ☐ relaxes
- ☐ gently stimulates nerve endings by clearing nerve pathways
- ☐ relieves tiredness and muscle pain.

ENDPOINTS
At the end of this topic you should understand:

- ☐ the movements and effects of effleurage
- ☐ the movements and effects of petrissage
- ☐ the movements and effects of tapotement
- ☐ the movements and effects of vibrations.

Topic 10:
The massage sequence

There are many different massage sequences. It is best to choose one of about 15 to 20 minutes which incorporates the face as well as the neck, shoulder and décolleté – which is where most clients hold tension – to practise and perfect the different movements and learn how to move smoothly from one movement to the next, before learning a new sequence. Once you can perform your massage efficiently you will learn to adapt the sequence to suit the needs of your client.

Contraindications

For general information on contraindications, see Chapter 1.
There are also some specific contraindications for massage treatment:

Contraindications requiring medical permission – in circumstances where medical permission cannot be obtained clients must give their informed consent in writing prior to the treatment

☐ Medical oedema	☐ Recent facial operations affecting the area	☐ Undiagnosed pain
☐ Nervous/Psychotic conditions		☐ When taking prescribed medication
☐ Epilepsy	☐ Skin cancer	
☐ Diabetes	☐ Slipped disc	☐ Whiplash

Contraindications that restrict treatment

☐ Fever	☐ Hormonal implants	☐ Recent fractures (minimum 3 months)
☐ Contagious or infectious diseases	☐ Sinusitis	
	☐ Neuralgia	☐ Trapped/pinched nerve affecting the treatment area
☐ Under the influence of recreational drugs or alcohol	☐ Sunburn	
	☐ Migraine/Headache	☐ Inflamed nerve
☐ Diarrhoea and vomiting	☐ Hypersensitive skin	
☐ Any known allergies	☐ Botox	If the contraindications are localised, it may be possible to avoid them during massage and continue with treatment. See Topic 8 for safety considerations when using massage oils and creams. In particular, be aware of any nut allergies if using nut-based products, such as almond oil, jojoba or arachis (peanut).
☐ Skin diseases	☐ Dermal fillers (1 week following treatment)	
☐ Undiagnosed lumps and bumps		
☐ Localised swelling	☐ Hyper-keratosis	
☐ Cuts, bruises, abrasions	☐ Skin allergies	
☐ Scar tissues (2 years for major operation and 6 months for a small scar)	☐ Inflammation	
	☐ Styes, watery eyes, eye infection, conjunctivitis, blepharitis	

Preparations for massage

Before starting the massage, prepare carefully to make the conditions as relaxing and stress free as possible.

Make sure:

- ☐ the room is warm and quiet
- ☐ you have everything you need easily to hand before you start
- ☐ your client is comfortable and warm
- ☐ you have warmed up your hands with finger and hand exercises

- ☐ the skin has been correctly prepared
- ☐ the massage medium is warmed
- ☐ you have covered any local areas of the face and neck contraindicated for massage
- ☐ you are in a comfortable position, at your client's head, that you can maintain for the whole massage either seated or standing.

During the massage

- ☐ Keep your movements flowing, rhythmical and unhurried.
- ☐ Be responsive and sensitive to the look and feel of your client's features and skin.

- ☐ Talk as little as possible but explain, when you think it necessary, what you are doing or about to do.
- ☐ Keep your hands in contact with your client's skin until the end of the massage.

A massage sequence

This sequence will cover your client's shoulders, neck, face and eye area and will include all the main classical massage movements. Here is an example sequence from an experienced practitioner.

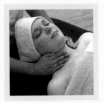 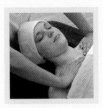 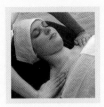 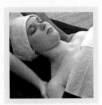 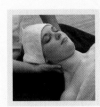

1. Effleurage starting at the mandible, down the platysma, across the pectorals, round the deltoids, trapezius and up in to the occipital bone to repeat, relieving tension along the trapezoid and in the neck area (occipitalis). Repeat six times.

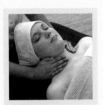 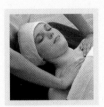 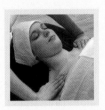 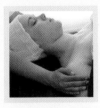 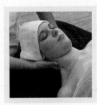

2. As above but rotate twice on the deltoid muscles. Repeat six times.

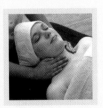 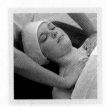 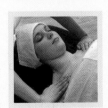 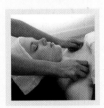 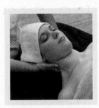

3. As above with the inclusion of knuckling along the pectorals. Repeat six times.

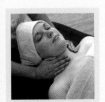 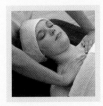 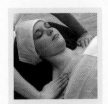 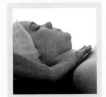 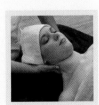

4. As above including thumb kneading along the trapezius and into the occipitalis. Repeat six times.

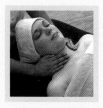 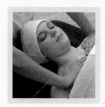 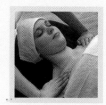 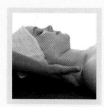 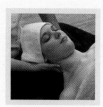

5. As overleaf but change to finger kneading along the trapezius and into the occipitalis Repeat six times.

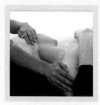

6. Stroking up either side of the neck. Turn the client's head over to the side. Deep effleurage up the side of the neck, then turn the client's head gently, place in position and stroke with alternate hands over the sternocleido-mastoid muscle up to the temporalis, and repeat. Always ensure that one hand is in contact with the skin before the other hand leaves. Good contact must not be broken Repeat six times.

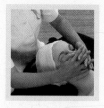 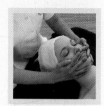 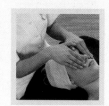 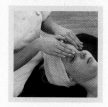 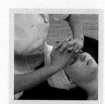 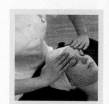

7. Face braces – do not drag the skin Repeat three times.

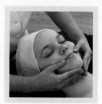 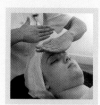 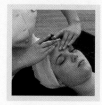 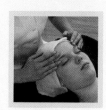

8. Flick ups Repeat three times.

9. Stroking very slowly along the whole forehead (frontalis) – side to centre, opposite side to centre.

10. Scissors on the forehead (frontalis) – side to centre, opposite side to centre

11. Stroking along the corrugators/eye brows Repeat six times.

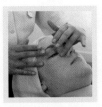 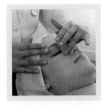 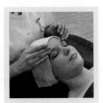

12. Half moons on the crows feet – do not drag the eye tissues. Repeat six times.

13. Stroking under the eye – do not drag the eye tissues Repeat six times.

14. Full eye circles Repeat six times.

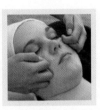 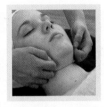 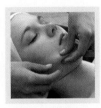 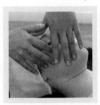 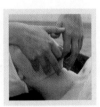

15. Knuckling on the cheeks

16. Knuckling along the mandible

17. Pincement in the mandible

18. Tapping along the mandible and cheeks

19. Tapping along the cheeks

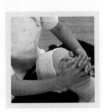 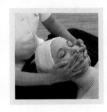 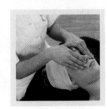 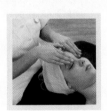 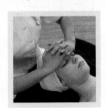 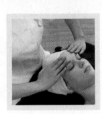

20. Face brace Repeat six times.

21. Repeat points 1–5

22. Finish with a vibration in the occipital area.

Topic 11: Masks

Clay masks

Clay-based masks are prepared by mixing the dry powder with a variety of active ingredients to form a smooth, easy-to-apply paste. Distilled (purified) water may be added to dilute the paste if a more liquid consistency is desired.

Clay masks can be individually mixed to benefit a range of skin types and requirements. Both the clays and the active ingredients have a variety of cleansing, toning, refining and stimulating effects so the constituents, and their proportions in a mask can be varied to create products with many different overall effects.

Clay ingredients and their effects

- **Calamine** – soothes inflamed skin and reduces vascularity; suitable for sensitive skin

- **Kaolin** – deep cleanses, removes impurities, stimulates circulation, helps desquamation and improves skin function, tightening the pores. Suitable for oily, congested skin

- **Magnesium carbonate** – mildly astringent, refines skin with open pores, stimulates to tighten and firm skin; suitable for young skin, or mixed with calamine for drier, more sensitive skins

- **Fuller's earth** – fast, strong action on blood circulation, excellent desquamation and deep cleansing; ideal for oily, congested skin, not suitable for sensitive skin

- **Flowers of sulphur** – very strong drawing, drying effect, dissolves surface dead skin cells, generally added to Fuller's earth for use on extremely oily skin.

Active ingredients and their effects

These should be matched to the clays for the appropriate skin type. While it is not itself an active ingredient, distilled water forms a perfect carrier for active ingredients, and its purity makes it less likely to irritate a sensitive skin. Active ingredients include:

- **Rosewater** – mildly toning effect, for mature, dry and sensitive skins

- **Orange flower water** – mildly toning effect, suitable for all skin types.

- **Witch hazel** – an astringent, drying and stimulating effect, for oily skin

- **Glycerine** – soothing and moisturising, for dry and dehydrated skin, a humectant which helps keep mask soft

- **Almond oil** – slightly stimulating and nourishing, helps hydration of dry skin.

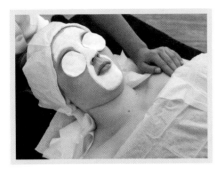 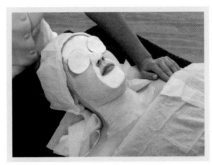 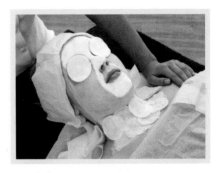

Applying clay masks

1. Apply lip balm to the lips and apply eye gel around the eyes.

2. Use a mask brush to apply the paste thinly, quickly and evenly on the skin. Use long strokes. The fewer the strokes the more even the mask.

3. If using one mask, apply the mask in sequence:

   – on the neck

   – the chin

   – one cheek, then the other cheek

   – the forehead.

4. When using more than one mask at a time, apply the mask to the area needing most treatment first (usually the T zone), so that it has maximum time on the skin.

5. Avoid the eyes, nostrils, mouth and eyebrows.

6. Apply cucumber to the eyes or eye pads soaked in cooling eye lotion if desired.

KEY POINT

Always stay with the client while the mask is on, in case of anxiety or skin reaction, so that you could remove the mask promptly if necessary.

Removing clay masks

1. Remove the mask when it is dry – for most masks 8 to 10 minutes is adequate, though some can be left on for 15 minutes.

2. If using more than one mask, remove them at the same time.

3. You can pre-moisten the mask to make it easier to remove by holding damp sponges over the set mask.

4. Remove the mask gently with warm water and sponges or cotton wool, changing the water when appropriate.

5. Make sure all traces of the mask are removed before treating with a toner and appropriate moisturiser.

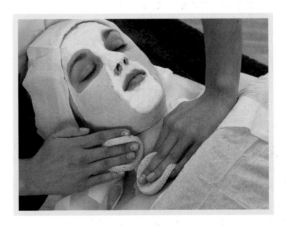

Natural or biological masks

Masks using natural products are simple but effective as plant enzymes can trigger reactions even in the deepest layers of the skin's cells. Natural masks are made from:

- fruit
- plants
- herbs
- natural products, such as eggs, yoghurts and honey, oatmeal.

Natural ingredients and their effects

- **Avocado** – very gentle on skin, with natural vitamins and minerals; its natural oil is beneficial for dry, mature or sensitive skins

- **Egg white** – has a toning and tightening effect, best for young or oily skin types; helps removal of comedones and other impurities; not recommended for dry or sensitive skins (adding lemon juice increases refining action and refines open pores)

- **Honey** – used to remove impurities and dead skin cells; lightens and hydrates skin, delaying formation of lines; all skin types

- **Banana** – contains potassium, calcium, phosphates and vitamins; good for dry and sensitive skins

- **Cucumber** – cooling effect; good for all skin types

- **Soft fruits**, such as strawberries, have an acid reaction on skin (can be mixed with yoghurt, cream or egg white to lessen acidic reaction), correct the pH balance of dry skin and increase moisture level

- **Natural yoghurt** – makes a very good base for masks

- **Lemon juice** – very stimulating; helps dry oily skin

- **Oatmeal** – good for desquamation

- **Egg yolk** – nourishes the skin; best for dry skins

- **Marine products** – hydrate and stabilise the skin

- **Herbs** – tone, stimulate, balance and regenerate; good for all skin types.

Natural masks and different skin types

As can be seen from the list above, natural masks can be made up to suit and benefit almost all skin types. They can be a useful alternative when treatments using chemicals or with alcohol-based products have been contraindicated for sensitive, mature or dry skins.

Hypersensitive skin conditions – natural masks can freshen and refine the skin gently while keeping the acid/alkali balance and improving cell renewal.

Dehydrated and dry skin conditions – natural masks can stimulate without further loss of moisture, leaving the skin fresh and soft with a fine texture and cleansed of dead skin cells.

Mature skins – natural masks' active ingredients help regeneration without irritating or reducing moisture.

Oily, blemished skins – natural masks deep cleanse and desquamate, removing oil, adhesions and bacteria from the skin's surface.

Suggestions for natural mask recipes

As with clay masks, there are many combinations of products that you can use to create different beneficial effects for different skin types. Here are a few examples:

For sensitive skin – yoghurt based

For dry skin – mash half a banana with ground almonds and olive oil

For oily skin – whisk together one egg white and a few drops of lemon juice

For oily or congested skin – mix salt, olive oil and juice of half a lemon; rub it over the skin gently with fingertips

Application and removal of natural masks

Because of their consistency, some natural masks may be more easily applied and removed between two layers of gauze.

1. Create your natural mask recipe with fresh ingredients just before you need to use it.

2. Place a layer of gauze over your client's face, with a hole cut out for the nose and mouth.

3. Cover your client's eyes with damp eye pads to stop any of the paste getting into the eyes.

4. Brush the paste over the neck and face area covered with gauze, avoiding the nostrils, eyes and mouth.

5. If necessary, cover the paste with another layer of gauze to keep it in place.

6. Leave the mask on for up to 20 minutes depending on the skin's reaction and the type of mask being used. As with clay masks, do not leave your client during this time and keep checking that she is comfortable with the mask on.

7. Remove the mask gently with luke-warm water and damp cotton wool pads or sponges.

8. When removal is complete, apply toner and moisturiser to suit your client's skin type.

Commercial masks

There are many types of commercially prepared masks available for all skin types. It is important to know the ingredients in any mask you use and make sure it is suitable for your client's skin type. You should also read and follow the manufacturer's instructions carefully, for the most effective way to use their products.

Specialised masks

There are a number of specialised masks whose ingredients have particular effects.

Thermal/mineral masks

Thermal masks work with an underlying cream or oil. This produces heat, which helps the skin absorb the creams. The cream chosen must be suitable to both the client's skin and the mask, so it is important to analyse the skin carefully first and, if necessary, use different creams for different areas of the face and neck.

Contraindications

See Chapter 1 for general contraindications to treatments, but specific contraindications to thermal masks are:

☐ highly strung clients

☐ clients with high vascular complexions.

Benefits of thermal masks

Thermal masks can benefit many different skin types according to the creams, used but in general they:

☐ are a very relaxing treatment

☐ stimulate the skin

☐ hydrate and tone the skin

☐ ease fine lines

☐ improve cellular regeneration.

Using thermal masks

1. Apply the cream to the face, leaving the eyes nostrils and mouth free.

2. Mix the thermal mask in accordance with the manufacturer's instructions, then apply as a thick paste over the cream.

3. Check that the paste is evenly distributed.

4. Cover your client's eyes with cotton wool pads and check she is comfortable.

5. Stay with the client as the mask hardens and then gradually subsides, usually about 20-30 minutes. Explain to your client that the mask will begin to feel heavy and will cool into a solid piece.

6. Remove the eye pads.

7. Remove the mask in one piece.

8. Do not dispose of any unused paste down a sink as it will harden and block pipes. Allow it to harden in the bowl and then dispose of it as a solid piece in a waste bin.

Peel-off masks

Peel-off masks form a sealing layer over the skin preventing moisture loss. They work by intensifying the penetration of an underlying cream. They are based on gels, latex or plastic resins and have a milder effect than clay masks as they are not absorbent. They peel off in one piece taking with them surface dirt and dead skin cells. They can be suitable for most skin types.

Benefits of peel-off masks

Gelling agents in gel masks can be mixed with many active ingredients, such as seaweed, aloe, camphor or ginseng, to benefit different skin types. Benefits of gel masks are that they:

☐ are mildly astringent

☐ soothe, calm and cool the skin

☐ moisturise and tighten the skin

☐ reduce the appearance of fine lines and wrinkles

☐ tend to be particularly suitable for mature and sensitive skins.

Latex masks:

☐ temporarily tighten the skin

☐ can be used to stimulate the blood supply

☐ are particularly suitable for dry and mature skins.

Using peel-off masks

Gel masks can be available in ready-mixed gel form or pellets which need heating before application. They are applied with a brush or spatula in an even layer over the face and neck. Follow the instructions for applying clay masks.

Latex masks can be applied in pre-cut shapes.

Peel-off masks, as their name implies, are designed to be gently peeled off the skin in one piece.

Collagen masks

Collagen masks come in two forms – as a paste to be mixed before application or for application as a sheet. Always consult the product instructions before use and follow the manufacturer's recommendations for application. The following is a typical sequence:

☐ Remove make-up.

☐ Cleanse face and rinse well.

☐ Lightly massage face for 5 to 8 minutes.

☐ Cover entire face with a warm towel and leave in place for 2 to 3 minutes, and then:

   – For a sheet mask, unfold the sheet and apply to face, using a gentle massage to forehead, nose and cheeks

   – For a mixed mask, apply in a thin layer over face and neck.

☐ Avoid direct contact with the eyes and do not drag delicate skin.

☐ Leave mask on for 15 to 30 minutes as specified by manufacturer.

☐ Gently remove mask following manufacturer's recommendations.

☐ Finish with toner and appropriate treatment for the client's skin type.

Hot oil masks

These masks combine the therapeutic effects of the underlying oil – such as arachis, olive or almond – with those of infra-red heat.

Contraindications

See Chapter 1 for general information on contraindications. In addition, there are specific contraindications for hot oil treatments:

☐ very nervous, highly strung clients

☐ hypersensitive skins

☐ high coloured complexions.

Areas of dilated capillaries must be covered with damp cotton-wool pads to prevent heat penetration.

Benefits of hot oil masks

Hot oil masks are used to:

☐ improve elasticity, smoothness and softness in dry, dehydrated and mature skins

☐ improve colour and skin tone.

Preparing for the hot oil mask

Place a piece of gauze soaked in the chosen oil in a small bowl inside a larger bowl of warm water in order to warm it prior to application to the client's skin.

Pre-heat an infra-red lamp away from the client checking that there are no trailing or loose wires, and that the lamp canopy is not dented. The lamp must be checked to ensure that is well balanced and will not fall.

1. After cleansing the skin, tone to ensure it is grease free.

2. Protect your client's hair and clothing with towels and paper tissues.

3. Shape a piece of gauze to suit your client's face and neck, with holes cut out for the nostrils and mouth.

4. Place eye pads over the eyes for protection.

Safety

Perform a thermal heat sensitivity test (see Chapter 8, Topic 4, page 262) before applying a hot-oil mask.

Using the hot oil mask

1. Place the gauze carefully over the clients face and neck.

2. Place the infra-red lamp in a stable position above the client's face, and at a minimum distance of 18 cms from the highest point (nose). Always follow the manufacturer's instructions for heat levels, distance and the sensitivity of your client's skin.

3. Do not leave the client.

4. Check your client's tolerance levels and comfort at regular intervals.

5. The procedure should take between 8 and 20 minutes depending upon the client's skin type and depth of treatment required.

6. Remove the lamp first and place it well away from the client, ensuring there are no trailing wires.

7. Remove the gauze and massage any remaining oil into the skin.

8. A mild, refreshing lotion can then be applied to the skin, followed by a protective moisturiser.

Record card

Remember, for all treatments, to note carefully on your client's record card exactly what treatments and products you have used and any reactions to these. For more information on filling out client record cards, see Chapter 1.

ENDPOINTS

You should now understand:

☐ the contraindications to mask use

☐ how to select the appropriate mask for the client's skin type

☐ clay masks

☐ natural masks

☐ commercial masks

☐ specialised masks.

Chapter 4: Using make-up

introduction

Using make-up is an ancient art, for which both the Egyptians and the Romans were famous. Many of the principles and some of the products they used are similar to those in use today, although scientific advances in cosmetics have greatly increased the possibilities and the safety factors.

A successful make-up session combines:

☐ good communication with your client – you must know what they want in order to achieve it for them

☐ careful analysis of your client's skin and facial structure

☐ a wide-ranging knowledge of the products available, their properties and effects

☐ a knowledge of how lighting, heat and time of day affect the look of make-up

☐ skilful application of the different products.

Topic 1: Communicating with your client

In order to achieve the required result, it is important to communicate effectively with your client throughout the application of make-up. Chapter 1 introduced you to professional ways of asking questions and listening to your client. With these in mind, we shall now look at the particular communication necessary for a successful make-up session.

What you need to find out

Why has the client chosen to have a make-up?

Be aware that, while some reasons for wanting a professional make-up session might be fun, routine or professional, others might be more personal and sensitive, so it is important to be sensitive in your reactions to what your client is telling you. Do they want the make-up:

☐ for a special occasion, e.g. a wedding, evening event, photographic shoot

☐ to learn how to apply her own make-up

☐ as part of a pampering session.

Finding out the particular reason will give you a good idea where to start:

☐ If it's for a wedding, then the make-up will often have to be suitable for both day and evening and have to match the colours of an outfit.

☐ An evening event or a photographic shoot may have to take into consideration either low or very bright, hot lighting.

☐ Corrective treatment will usually need to rely more on concealing make-up with the emphasis on a natural look.

☐ Your client may just want to know how to accentuate their best features (and minimise the others) and be relying completely on you to advise them.

Do they have a particular look in mind?

Your client may know exactly what they want, and even have a picture to show you. It is important to be aware of modern fashions in make-up (which can sometimes change quite rapidly) as well as classic looks. They might have favourite colours or know what they want accentuated. They may only have a vague idea in which case they will be relying heavily on you and your ideas and guidance.

Your client, contraindications and the record card

Your client may be able to tell you about any possible contraindications, such as allergies to particular products, and it is important to ask and note anything down on the record card for future treatments.

ENDPOINTS
You should now understand:

☐ what the therapist needs to find out from the client

☐ the importance of maintaining appropriate records.

Topic 2: Preparing for make-up

Before applying make-up, it is very important to recognise your client's skin type and to prepare the skin accordingly. Chapter 3 Topic 2 explains how to analyse your client's skin, thoroughly observing it through a magnifying lamp after thorough cleansing, and how to complete the client's record card, using initial observation, touch and effective communication (see also Chapter 1)

Knowing your client's skin

By the time you have completed a full skin analysis, you will have an individual picture of your client's skin and the conditions that affect it. You will also be able to choose products that are appropriate to your individual client.

Skin types and characteristics

There are a range of skin types, each with its own particular characteristics. Both the skin colour, which can vary from pale white to various shades of black, and the evenness of colour will affect and be an indicator of the skin's sensitivity to a range of factors and external stimuli such as ageing, exposure to UV radiation, hydration, facial hair growth and skin blemishes.

Production of the pigment melanin varies according to skin type and characteristics. Black skins contain no more melanocytes than white, but the melanin granules in black skin are larger and hence more obvious.

Here are the main skin types and characteristics:

☐ **White skin** – fair in colour, often with freckles and accompanied by red, blonde or brown hair and green/blue eyes. Tends to be more sensitive to UV rays and external stimuli, to age more quickly and show vascular disorder, for instance in a florid complexion. Because white skin ages more quickly than black, it is important to start protecting the skin from UV rays as early as possible

☐ **Black skin** – produces a large amount of melanin which determines the skin colour and depth. Although varying greatly in shades, black skin generally has greater protection from damaging UV rays, tends to be more supple with delayed ageing effects, but more reactive to stimuli such as rashes or inflammations which can leave dark marks and scarring on the skin. It is also more prone to keloid scarring. It is generally oily skin, but if it becomes dry, dead skin cells appear ashen.

☐ **Asian-type skin** – predominantly yellow in tone with a sallow tinge. It is often oily but smooth and evenly coloured. Asian skin ages very well and does not suffer with the many lines and wrinkles that tend to affect white skins, but is more prone to hyperpigmentation from operation scars and lesions, so should be treated with care.

☐ **Mixed skin** – a combination of all or some of the skin types; the shades and sensitivities will vary greatly depending upon the mix.

☐ **Dry skin** – generally appears pale and thin, with fine lines, no visible pores, sometimes broken capillaries and flakiness, and may feel and look tight. It may be a result of dehydration, and, although more commonly associated with middle age, it can appear at any age and be caused by genetic, internal or external factors, such as suntanning. Treatments stimulate the dry skin to correct the oil and moisture balance.

☐ **Oily skin** – may appear sallow and dull or shiny and hard (seborrhoea), with uneven texture and enlarged pores, particularly down the central T zone, with comedones (black heads) and papules.

Due to an over-secretion of the sebaceous glands, often during adolescence and frequently affected by the menstrual cycle, it can occur at any time in areas of the face. Generally, treatments seek to unblock pores through specialised cleaning routines, but must avoid dehydrating the skin with harsh products.

☐ **Combination skin** – Can be a combination of any two skin types on the same face although there is generally a central oily zone, with the cheeks and neck showing normal or dry skin. This is a very common skin type, and there are now products created specially for combination skin types.

☐ **Mature skin** – with age, the skin will lose firmness and elasticity, and may feel looser and thinner, although the hormonal changes of the menopause may cause thickening on the chin. This change in texture may cause the appearance of fine lines, and less definition of the contours of the face. As the sebaceous glands become less active, the skin becomes drier. The skin appears thinner – almost transparent in areas such as those surrounding the eyes, where small capillaries may show through the skin. Waste products are removed more slowly from a mature skin, leading to puffiness, particularly around the eyes. The surface of the skin may begin to display areas of irregular pigmentation in the form of lentigo or chloasma.

☐ **Young skin** – looks even in colour, with fine, clear texture, soft, smooth and supple but firm, with a balance of oil and moisture. This, rather rare, type generally only needs protection and maintenance treatment.

Skin conditions and texture

Blemished skin tends to feel coarse and bumpy and may indicate present or previous skin conditions. Skin conditions and textures include:

☐ **dehydrated skin** – skin that has lost water from the tissues. The skin will show fine superficial lines, and superficial flaking and broken capillaries may occur. This affects all skin types, and may be related to the clients' general health, lifestyle, diet or skin care regime. In many cases it is caused by a working environment that is air-conditioned or low in humidity

☐ **lack of elasticity** – which may be evident as lines that appear around the eyes and mouth. Oily skins may age better than dry skins, but often suffer more blemishes, particularly during puberty

☐ **lack of muscle tone** – dropped facial contours usually indicate a mature skin whose muscles are becoming slacker with age

☐ **blemishes** – are temporary or permanent marks on the skin, including broken capillaries, comedones, milia, papules, pustules, scarring moles and pigmentation spots

☐ **age** – as the skin ages there may appear to be loss of tone in the facial expression muscles, more prominent bones, fine wrinkling around the eyes, generally finer and less elastic skin, which is looser on the neck and eyelids, may show broken capillaries on the cheeks and nose, and in which pigmentation is becoming more evident

☐ **crows feet** – fine lines around the eyes caused by habitual expressions and daily movement, associated with ageing of muscle tissue. Premature formation may be due to eye strain and is often associated with oedema (swelling) around and under the eyes

☐ **comedones** – commonly known as blackheads, these are caused by a build-up of sebaceous secretions which have become trapped in the hair follicles and have subsequently dried out and hardened. The colour comes from oxidation. Common in puberty

☐ **milia** – commonly known as whiteheads, these form when sebum becomes trapped in a blind duct with no surface opening. The condition is most common on dry skin and milia appear on the obicularis oculi muscle area and between the eyebrows

☐ **pustules** – a small inflamed elevation of the skin filled with fluid or pus

☐ **papules** – a small, solid, unusually inflammatory elevation of the skin that does not contain pus

☐ **ingrowing hairs** – when hairs begin to regrow, particularly after shaving or waxing, they may double over on themselves and curl up inside the hair follicle, as they are unable to exit the surface. The hair continues to grow inside the foillicle, triggering a foreign body reaction, which causes inflammation and a red bump on the surface of the skin

☐ **open pores** – due to oily skin or, in a mature client with dry skin, due to a previous skin condition

□ **sensitive skin** – can look like dry skin, usually with high colour, or warmth in darker skin, with signs of dilated capillaries. It is easily stimulated, often becoming red and blotchy, and responds quickly to treatment, so care is needed. Treatments emphasise calming routines and products to maintain the skin's balance

□ **broken capillaries** (couperose) – indicating sensitive or thin skin

□ **hypo pigmentation** – darker pigmented areas possibly indicating sun damage

□ **hyper pigmentation** – uneven patches of skin tone, lighter than the surrounding skin due to lack of melanin in the area

□ **dermatosis papulosa nigra** – also called flesh moles, these are brown or black hyper pigmentation markings resembling moles. The cause is unknown but sometimes found to be hereditary. It most frequently occurs on female black skin

□ **pseudo folliculitis** – an inflammatory skin disorder which mainly occurs in male black skins as the hair is coarser and curly and has a tendency as it grows out for the skin to curl back and re-enter the follicle becoming ingrowing making the skin irritated and inflamed. Hyper pigmentation may also accompany this condition

□ **keloids** – scarring that becomes enlarged and projects from the skin's surface, caused by hyperpasia

□ **scarring** – due to injury, chickenpox or post acne

□ **thin skin** – due, for instance, to steroid treatment for severe eczema

□ **small raised moles** (benign melanomas) or birthmarks.

Skin tones

In addition to the characteristics and conditions listed above, a client's skin may be classified by tone as one of either:

□ fair

□ medium

□ dark

□ olive

Preparing your client's skin

Chapter 3 took you through the stages of cleansing and toning your client's skin, from the initial cleanse to various deep cleansing treatments. It is important always to prepare your client's skin before applying make-up.

Cleansing

The initial cleanse is essential to remove any previous make-up and superficial dirt, and to find out the immediate condition of the client's skin. Correct preparation of the skin greatly aids the longevity of the make-up. If there is time, a deep cleanse may also be included before make-up, but check that it is appropriate to apply make-up after the treatment that you and your client have chosen. It is preferable to leave the skin clear from make-up for as long as possible after a facial treatment.

Using moisturiser

After the skin has been cleansed and toned, it should be moisturised before applying make-up. Moisturisers are necessary in order to:

□ combat the drying effects of the environment (central heating, sun, wind, etc.)

□ replenish the skin's moisture levels, which may be reduced by astringent products used on the skin, or the ageing process

□ act as a barrier between skin and make-up

□ keep the skin supple and smooth

□ act as a sun screen (many moisturisers now contain UVA and UVB sunblocks, and are available with a range of sun protection factors, or SPFs – which should be a minimum of 15 in normal day creams)

□ provide a smooth base for foundation.

Moisturising products

As with any other skin creams and lotions, it is important to use a moisturiser that is appropriate to the skin type and condition. Moisturisers are emulsions in the form of creams or liquids (milks) which vary the oil to water ratio to suit different skins. They generally contain a humectant, such as glycerine, to attract and hold moisture in the skin. However, if the air is very dry, moisturiser should be frequently replenished to keep the skin moist obviously this would not be possible if make-up was being worn. Clients may need to use higher performance products depending upon the environment and climatic conditions where they live, and their age.

Moisturising creams – have a higher oil to water ratio, which prevents water escaping from the skin. Creams are now available that are appropriate for all skin types, but they are particularly suitable for:

☐ clients with dry skins (the cream acts as an emollient)

☐ clients living or working in very dry atmospheres, e.g. air-conditioned offices

☐ mature clients.

Moisturising liquids (milks) – have a higher water to oil ratio, adding water to the skin and attracting it from the atmosphere. They are lighter and more absorbent than creams, and do not leave a greasy film on the skin. They are particularly suitable for:

☐ rehydrating a dehydrated skin

☐ oily skins.

Night creams – are generally much richer and heavier than day creams and are sometimes used for more mature skins. Due to the consistency of the creams it is difficult to add SPFs which is why day creams must be worn in the day with the SPF. Night time is when the skin naturally renews itself as the body rests, hence the use of a deeper treatment cream at night.

Tinted moisturisers – may be used instead of a foundation, especially for clients with clear skins.

ENDPOINTS
You should now understand how:

☐ clients' skin types may vary

☐ to prepare the client's skin

☐ to use moisturiser.

Topic 3:
The make-up chart

After finding out what your client wants and analysing their skin, you can draw up a make-up plan. The make-up plan is a record of what you are going to do and why, and the products you are going to use. You should take into consideration:

☐ the occasion

☐ the lighting

☐ the client's skin type, colouring, face shape and features.

To do this, your client should be sitting comfortably to ensure the facial contours are as they would normally be in an evenly lit room in front of a mirror with as natural lighting as possible – daylight or white fluorescent light is best. If the client were lying down the facial contours would not be representative and this might affect the outcome of the make-up application.

The occasion

Daytime – A natural look is usually preferred for daytime make-up, enhancing your client's natural colours and best features. It is also the time that will show up your technique most, as harsh lines or contrasts between colours will appear stark and unnatural unless carefully applied.

Weddings – As for daytime, only more so! As well as make-up that will look good close up in natural light and in photographs (pearlised make-up will reflect in photographs), it must also go well with the hairstyle, clothes and colour scheme of the day (bridesmaids' dresses, bouquets). In most cases, it must also last through to the evening, which would suggest the use of a double layer of lipstick with a layer of powder in between. In this situation, your client will greatly benefit from your advice on how to:

☐ turn a day make-up quickly and effectively into an evening make-up

☐ prolong the longevity of the make-up.

Wedding make-up requires careful planning and a trial session before the day to decide on products and effects and to plan timing. You should also give advice on how to refresh and prolong the make-up, such as carrying a spare lipstick and face powder. Waterproof mascara is a good idea for an emotional occasion!

Evenings – Colours and techniques should be adapted for artificial light, low lighting, such as candle light, or coloured lighting. In general, this means adding and emphasising colours and definition and, depending on the occasion, adding gloss and sparkle. Make-up should still be applied in clear, white light.

Photographic – As for evening make-up, the colours and definition should be more dramatic and bolder, as bright photographic lighting can whiten out colour and effects. However, it can also cruelly show up blemishes, which will need to be carefully concealed. Depending on the purpose of the shoot, the make-up should either try to recreate a natural look, or should be deliberately bold in its final effect. Pearlised make-up should be used carefully as it can be reflective in photographs.

Make-up lesson – If your client wants to learn how to apply their own make-up at home, then it is important to discuss with them at every stage what you are doing and why. Tell them about the products best suited to their skin condition and colouring, and show how to use them and how to enhance their best features while minimising those they are not so happy with. This should be a very positive experience for your client.

Camouflage make-up – this is applied to cover major skin imperfections, such as pigmentation disorders, birthmarks, tattoos, burns and scarring. Use special camouflage make-up, which should generally be waterproof, sunproof, hypo-allergenic and match your client's skin colour exactly (you may have to mix colours to achieve this). Be sensitive to your client's needs and fears and be positive in your approach; teaching clients how to apply the products themselves should help give them more confidence, especially when they see the end results. See page 145 for how to apply corrective make-up. Be aware of any doctor's recommendations and be especially careful when filling in your client's record card.

Client's skin type and characteristics

Your client's colouring will greatly affect the products you use and the final look. Remind yourself of the basic skin colours and their characteristics (see Chapter 3, Topic 2) and also that there are graduations in colour in every skin type from palest white to deep blue-black. While you will need to adjust the colours and products you use to your individual client's colouring, skin and characteristics, there are some general points to be aware of.

- On white skin, even pale colours will show up easily.

- For white-skinned people, the colouring of the hair and eyes is as important as the tones of the skin when choosing make-up colours. For instance, white skinned people with dark hair and eyes will generally suit darker make-up colours better than those with lighter hair and blue eyes.

- On black skin, foundation with cover can have a dulling effect, so it should be transparent, or you could use a coloured gel or tinted moisturiser instead; similarly, either use a translucent face powder or none at all.

- Black skins with uneven pigmentation (patchy colouring or much darker colouring, for instance underneath the eyes) will need concealer, but this should not be too light or it will create too great a contrast with the natural skin colour.

- On olive and black skins, colours should be darker and more intense to have an effect.

- While all make-up colours should be tried out on each individual client's skin, to match actual tones, make-up colours applied directly onto black skin may appear very different, so extra care should be taken. For instance, it may be advisable to put a light or grey undercoat of eye shadow as a neutral base for the true colour of the eye shadow to come through. However, there are many ranges of make-up now designed especially for black skins, which take this into consideration.

- Asian skin types, with yellow undertones, need foundation with a yellow base.

- On darker skin colours, it is not always easy to see whether an allergic reaction has been produced. You need to be very attentive to this and note your client's skin temperature and whether she feels any discomfort. If in any doubt, use hypo-allergenic products.

Face shapes

Faces come in all sorts of individual shapes but are most often sorted into seven archetypal groups: oval, square, heart-shaped, oblong (long), diamond-shaped, pear-shaped and round. Using these as patterns will generally determine where you will place the three main shaping tools of make-up:

☐ highlighter

☐ blusher

☐ shader.

This type of make-up is sometimes known as corrective, as it attempts to 'correct' the face shape to resemble the oval.

☐ Many regard the oval as the most desirable shape although, as with everything, there are fashions and cultural differences in desirable face shapes.

☐ However, the effects that using shader, highlighter and blusher create are generally agreed. Your client's face shape and features, and how your client feels about them, will largely determine the way you apply her make-up; that is, which parts of the face you highlight and which you shade.

☐ Remember that highlighter draws the features forward, whilst shader draws the features back.

☐ Apply shader to areas you want to draw attention away from, such as the chin in long faces or the sides of the jaw in pear-shaped, square or round faces.

☐ Apply highlighter to those areas where you want to give the illusion of width or length, as down the centre of a round face, or to the sides of the temples and lower jaw in a diamond-shaped face.

☐ Apply blusher to enhance the bone structure in most faces, high on the cheekbones in round or pear-shaped faces, and on the fullness of the cheeks in oblong, diamond-shaped and heart-shaped faces.

☐ Alternatively, you can shape a face using blusher alone by:

– using it to shade the sides of the face to create the illusion of length

– using it on the cheeks, or angling it from the cheekbones to the ears, to create the illusion of width.

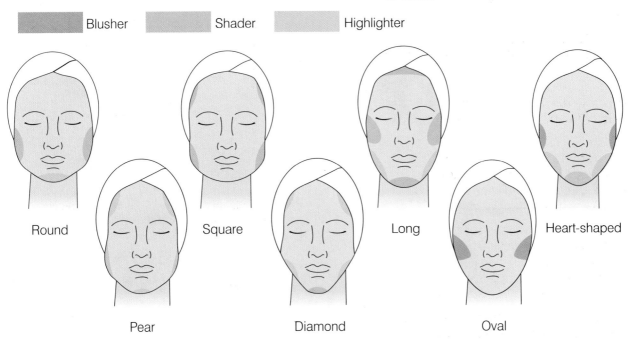

Blusher   Shader   Highlighter

Round   Square   Long   Heart-shaped

Pear   Diamond   Oval

Eye shapes

Eyes can be roughly categorised by their shape as, for instance, round or small, and by their position on the face, e.g. close-set. These categories will generally dictate the way make-up is applied to the eyes. Remember that darker shades draw the features back and highlighter draws the feature forward.

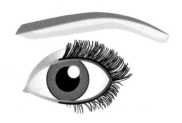

Make-up correction for small eyes

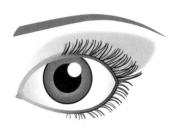

Make-up correction for close-set eyes

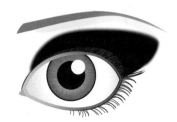

Make-up correction for prominent eyes

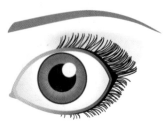

Make-up correction for round eyes

Small eyes – give the illusion of larger eyes by:

☐ arching the eyebrow and echoing it below with highlighter and dark shadow

☐ building up the eyelashes with mascara

☐ applying a thin sweeping eyeliner slightly above and below the eye line, not meeting at the outer edges

☐ applying a light colour to the lid, accentuating the central lid area with a more definite shade.

Close-set eyes – draw attention away from the centre of the face and towards the outer edges of the brows, lashes and eyelids by:

☐ creating a larger space between the brows (tweezing)

☐ using darker eye shadow, eye liner and mascara on the outer edges of the eyes

☐ filling in the rest of the lid and below the brow with a lighter shadow to emphasise space.

Prominent eyes – draw attention away from the eyes by:

☐ applying a darker shade to the upper lid, extending it slightly outwards

☐ emphasising the brow, tapering it and adding highlighter on the brow bones

☐ not emphasising the lashes.

Round eyes – add shape to the eyes by:

☐ extending eye shadow and eyeliner out beyond the outer corner of the eye

☐ highlighting the upper lid with a pale tone

☐ accentuating the arch of the brow from the centre to the outside edge with highlighter

☐ thickening the lashes from the centre to the outer edge.

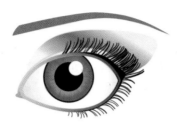

Make-up correction for dropping eyes

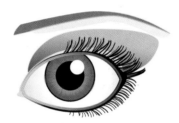

Make-up correction for hooded eyes

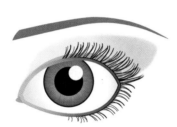

Make-up correction for deep-set eyes

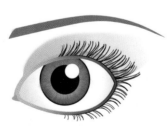

Make-up correction for wide-set eyes

Drooping eyes – eyes that droop downwards on the outer edges should be lifted by:

☐ blending darker shadow and eyeliner upwards and out from the centre and outside edge of the lid

☐ using lighter eye shadow on the inside edge of the lid

☐ using highlighter below the outside edge of the brow

☐ building up the top outer lashes with mascara.

Hooded eyes – should be lifted by:

☐ arching and tapering the brow and adding highlighter beneath it

☐ shading the overhanging skin with a deeper-toned shadow

☐ emphasising the eyes with darker eyeliner and mascara

☐ highlighting the upper lid with a light, possibly pearlised, eye shadow, which could be echoed with light shadow below the bottom lashes.

Deep-set eyes – to draw attention to the eyes, bringing them forward by:

☐ applying light coloured eye shadow all over the eyelids to accentuate the eyes

☐ slightly darker shade being applied to the outer corners blending upwards and outwards

☐ eyeliner applied to the outer halve of the upper and lower eyelids

Wide-set eyes – to draw attention towards the centre of the face and away from the outer edges of the brows, lashes and eyelids by

☐ applying darker eye shadow to the inner area of the eyelid and lighter eye shadow to the outer area of the eyelid

☐ using darker eye liner and mascara on the inner edges of the eyes

☐ using eyebrow pencil to extend the inner brow line

Large eyes – generally regarded as fine features that do not need 'correcting', but can be enhanced. See Topic 4: Applying eye make-up.

Lip shapes

Lips can be categorised roughly into:

- ☐ small/narrow/thin
- ☐ uneven/asymmetrical
- ☐ over large/full
- ☐ drooping.

Each size and shape will have its associated shaping and colouring make-up.

- ☐ Thin lips are increased in size by redrawing the lip line outside the natural line and filling in. Highlighter, darker colours and gloss can appear to give fullness to smaller lips.

- ☐ Over-large lips are decreased by blotting out the natural line with foundation and powder (unless having over-large lips is the fashion – in which case they are accentuated!). Use softer colours and a fairly matt lipstick, so as not to draw attention to them.

- ☐ Uneven/asymmetrical lips can be redrawn symmetrically.

- ☐ Drooping lips are lifted at the corners of the upper lip, while reshaping and blotting out the lower lip droop.

Block out the desired shape with foundation and powder first, before firming the outline with lipstick and lip line.

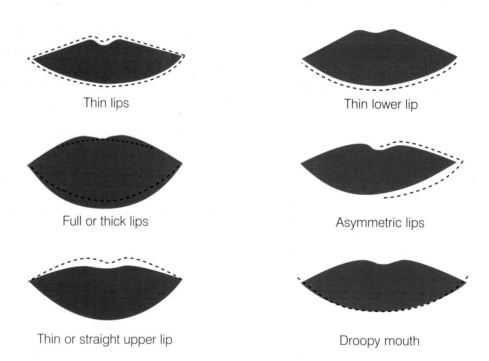

Thin lips

Thin lower lip

Full or thick lips

Asymmetric lips

Thin or straight upper lip

Droopy mouth

Corrective make-up for minor blemishes

Flaws such as dark circles under the eyes or spots do not need the specialist corrective and camouflage make-up necessary for burns and birthmarks, but do need treating separately before applying make-up in the normal manner. For:

☐ **high colour** – apply a green corrective cream and then foundation to disguise redness and broken capillaries

☐ **sallow skin** – apply lilac- corrective cream underneath foundation

☐ **dark circles under eyes and minor hyperpigmentation** – apply a light reflecting concealer or lighter foundation over dark areas (see also note about black skins, above)

☐ **puffy eyes** – use a darker shade of foundation on the bags and a lighter shade on the crease under the bags

☐ **isolated skin blemishes** – use cover sticks, creams or concealers in fair, medium and dark shades to blend in with foundation.

The whole face and the make-up plan

Features such as the eyes and lips should never be considered in isolation, but always in relation to each other and to the overall shape of the face and other features, such as the nose, ears, chin, hair and hairline. They should balance, complement, draw attention to or away from each other according to the desired effect. This is something you will learn to achieve with practice, but is an essential and enjoyable part of the art of make-up.

You can now fill in the complete make-up chart, which you will have explained to and agreed with your client.

Contraindications to make-up

Look back at Chapters 1, 2 and 3 to remind yourself about total contraindications, those with GP permission, localised contraindications, and specific contraindications to skin-care and eye treatments. In the main, contraindications also apply to make-up, but we shall add any further contraindications to specific techniques and products as they arise in this chapter.

As a quick reminder, the main contraindications to be aware of are:

Contraindications requiring medical permission – in circumstances where medical permission cannot be obtained clients must give their informed consent in writing prior to the treatment

☐ Medical oedema	☐ Diabetes	☐ When taking prescribed medication
☐ Nervous/Psychotic conditions	☐ Skin cancer	
☐ Epilepsy	☐ Slipped disc	☐ Whiplash
☐ Recent facial operations affecting the area	☐ Undiagnosed pain	

Contraindications that restrict treatment

☐ Fever	☐ Cuts, bruises, abrasions	☐ Botox
☐ Contagious or infectious diseases	☐ Scar tissues (2 years for major operation and 6 months for a small scar)	☐ Dermal fillers (1 week following treatment)
☐ Under the influence of recreational drugs or alcohol	☐ Sunburn	☐ Skin allergies
☐ Diarrhoea and vomiting	☐ Hormonal implants	☐ Styes, watery eyes, eye infection, conjunctivitis
☐ Any known allergies	☐ Recent fractures (minimum 3 months)	☐ Trapped/pinched nerve affecting the treatment area
☐ Eczema	☐ Sinusitis	
☐ Undiagnosed lumps and bumps	☐ Neuralgia	☐ Inflamed nerve
☐ Localised swelling	☐ Migraine/Headache	☐ Blepharitis
☐ Inflammation	☐ Hypersensitive skin	

ENDPOINTS

At the end of this section you should understand the implications for the type, design and performance of a make-up treatment of:

☐ the occasion

☐ the client's colouring

☐ face shapes

☐ eye shapes

☐ lip shapes

☐ considerations of corrective make-up for minor blemishes

☐ the relationship between the whole face and the make-up plan

☐ contraindications to make-up.

Topic 4: Applying make-up

As with all skin care products, you must select make-up products that match your client's skin type, colour and characteristics. Remind yourself of skin types and their characteristics and contraindications by looking at Chapter 3 and reread the notes on skin colour in this chapter.

Applying make-up properly requires technique and practice and knowledge of proper hygiene methods.

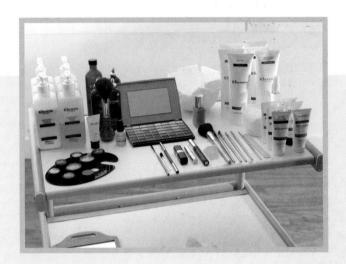

Preparing the working area

Remember to allow time between clients in which to check and prepare your working area. You should be aiming to tidy up after the previous client and treatment and prepare for the next client or treatment. To do this you need to:

☐   dispose of used preparations

☐   remove disposable tools (if used)

☐   sterilise or sanitise reusable tools

☐   set out sanitised tools

☐   set out preparations for the treatment

☐   perform your pre-client checklists (see Chapter 1).

As well as ensuring that the treatment room is well-lit, if the make-up is to include some client instruction you will need to make sure that mirrors are appropriately positioned and illuminated.

Preparing the client

The client's skin will need to be prepared for the make-up session.

Refer to Chapter 3 to ensure that appropriate skin analysis and cleansing preparations have been performed, and earlier topics in this chapter on preparation for make-up.

Pre-base creams

A pre-base cream is a light moisturising cream or lotion.

It forms an ideal base for an even foundation as it smoothes out the surface of the skin and helps minimise open pores, lines and wrinkles.

Correction creams

In texture, similar to moisturiser, these creams work on the complimentary colour theory, see below.

Colour correction creams help disguise skin blemishes and give an even tone to discoloured skins.

Complementary colours

The three primary colours (red, blue and yellow) each have a complementary secondary colour (green, orange and violet) which, when mixed together, neutralize them. Colour complementary theory is used extensively in make-up in concealing products and also for striking colour effects when the colours are put next to each other.

Foundation

The main purpose of foundation is to even out the skin's texture and colour, so that make-up can be applied to a consistent base to:

☐ moisturise

☐ provide a matt finish on oily skin

☐ cover minor blemishes

☐ brighten or enhance the complexion

Foundations come in:

☐ **liquids** – high water to oil ratio, suitable for oily skin, light film coverage; can be medicated with antiseptic

☐ **gels** – non greasy, jelly-like liquids; a thin film of colour suitable for smooth black and clear skins; give a natural tanned look to lighter skins

☐ **creams** – higher oil to water ratio, with powder and humectant; thicker and heavier; suitable for dry and mature skins; can appear to even out lines; need setting with loose powder

☐ **mousses** – give light cover; normally come in aerosols or dispensers

☐ **blocks/compacts/cakes** – convenient form of compressed cream and powder or more solid forms using wax; medium to heavy coverage; suitable for most skins, though dry skins should use the cream versions

☐ **all-in-one** – creams with powder; not suitable for dry or sensitive skins; leave a matt finish

☐ **light reflecting** – light reflecting foundations for mature skin, eyelids and lips

☐ **matt** – high water ratio, suitable for oily and combination skin.

Choosing foundation colours

As a general rule, foundation should match as closely as possible the existing skin tone. However, if it is used to enhance or neutralise skin tones, use:

☐ golden and tan shades to add warmth

☐ beige or orange shades to neutralise pink or red tones

☐ rose or bronze shades to brighten sallow or olive skins.

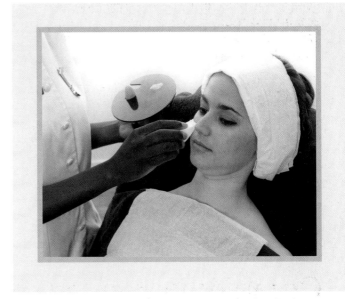

Contraindications

See general contraindications to skin care and make-up treatments on page 146.

Applying foundation

☐ Always decant enough foundation onto a palette first, using a clean spatula not your fingers.

☐ Use a damp sponge, make-up wedges or flat brushes or fingers to blend foundation

☐ Work quickly and lightly from the centre to the hairline, and below the jaw line to the neck.

☐ Be especially careful to blend the foundation into the creases around the nose and eyes.

☐ Cover the eyelids and lips as a base for longer lasting eye shadow and lipstick.

☐ The final look should be as natural and unobtrusive as possible.

Concealer

A good concealer will not only hide a spot or blemish – some will also dry it out. For black skins, choose an orange shade for darker areas and yellow for purple patches. Do not use a heavy concealer under the eyes, but instead use a light cream that is not too oily.

Depending on the condition to be covered, concealers come in:

☐ sticks or pots – thicker and opaque

☐ tubes, wands or pens – lighter, easier to blend, less opaque, for clients who wear little make-up.

Applying concealer

Test the colour first on your client's jaw line in daylight, to see whether it matches the skin tone. Apply using:

☐ wedge-shaped sponges for large areas, such as patches under the eyes

☐ cotton buds for small blemishes

☐ small bristle brushes for scars and fine lines.

Safety: to stop cross-infection, never apply sticks straight onto the skin. Scrape a little off the stick with a spatula or orange stick before applying.

Face powder

Face powder is used primarily to fix foundation, but it also:

☐ provides a suitable base for powder blushers and shaders

☐ removes shine, giving the skin a matt appearance by reflecting light

☐ helps conceal minor blemishes.

Face powder comes in two main forms.

☐ Loose – used by professionals:

   – translucent and light reflecting, with high proportions of kaolin and chalk

   – good coverage and sometimes coloured.

☐ Pressed – traditional retail powder:

   – not fine enough for professional use, contains wax or gum

   – good for touching up make-up or removing shine during the day.

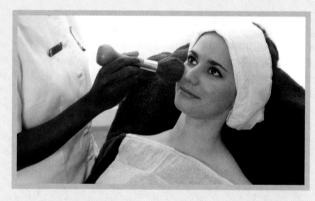

☐ Coloured powders

   – Coloured powder can appear unnatural and may change colour when in contact with oils from skin and can change foundation colour

   – Some powders can have silver or gold particles to add extra shine for evening wear, or bronze for a light golden look

   – Remember that a pearlised powder can be reflective in photographs

   – Translucent powder can leave a chalky effect on black skin, so brown, bronze or gold are preferable options.

Contraindications

Before applying face powder, remind yourself of any contraindications to using skin products.

Applying face powder

☐ First, make sure your client's eyes and mouth are closed.

☐ Decant the powder either on to a palette or onto a cotton wool pad

☐ Apply face powder using a cotton-wool pad or powder brush, tapping off excess first.

☐ Press on the foundation, covering all areas including eyelids and mouth.

☐ Brush off excess powder using a downward motion to ensure the powder does not stick in the facial hairs to leave skin smooth and even, with no extra particles in eyelashes or brows.

Safety:

to stop contamination decant the powder first and never put a used cotton-wool pad back into the powder container.

Contour cosmetics

Shaders, highlighters and blushers are known as contour cosmetics because they are used to accentuate, enhance and minimise features by emphasising and contouring the shapes of the face. We looked at how to do this in Topic 3.

Contraindications

As well as the general contraindications and those specifically for make-up, contour cosmetics should not be applied over crepey, lined or very hairy skin. In addition, dry, flaky skin is contraindicated for use with cosmetic powders.

They come in various forms.

☐ **Creams** – applied over foundation but before face powder; add moisture as well as colour

☐ **Gels** – applied over foundation but never covered with face powder; for a transparent, more natural look

☐ **Sticks** – applied over foundation; difficult to blend thoroughly

☐ **Powders** – applied after face powder; blend well; smooth finish; more appropriate for evening, fashion and photographic make-up.

Shaders

Shaders should be darker than the foundation colour to be effective, but not so dark as to appear unnatural, as very warm, dark colours can sometimes appear orange and then act as blusher rather than shader.

Highlighters

Highlighters should be lighter than the foundation colour to emphasise bone structure and draw attention to eyes and cheekbones. They can also help to hide deep lines.

Eye shadow

Eyes are generally regarded as the most important and expressive features and the main focus of attention, so it is not surprising that eye make-up is often regarded as the most important. It is also the most artistic. Eye shadow, of all the eye make-ups, is the most colourful, so it is used not just to match the skin but to enhance beauty and complement eye colour and often clothes and jewellery. It comes in several forms.

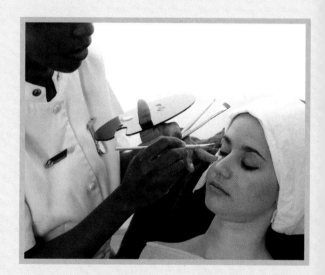

- ☐ **Cream** – oil-based; spreads easily, but needs powder to set and tends to crease – this is not recommended for mature clients

- ☐ **Powders** – creamy powder with oil; pressed or loose, matt, can have pearlised, metallic or frosted effects; less suitable for dry skins.

- ☐ **Water colours** – cake eye shadow applied with wet brush; strong colour, long lasting.

- ☐ **Pencils** – oil or wax based; easy to apply; can give hard lines or be blended in.

Colours

An almost endless variety of colours can be achieved using contrasting and complementary colours in eye shadow. Earlier, we looked at using eye shadow to enhance and 'correct' the shape of the eye, but it can also be used to enhance the eye colour, create fashion or photographic effects, mix and match with accessories, or just for fun. Your client may prefer particular shades, or she may take your advice, so it is good to familiarise yourself with a range of effects using different colours and techniques. These are some suggestions for starting points.

- ☐ Darker browns and reds can subtly enhance dark eyes.

- ☐ Pastel colours enhance light grey, green or blue eyes.

- ☐ Very light colours create highlights when used with darker eye shadow.

- ☐ Bright colours are best for young, fun, fashion looks.

- ☐ Softer greys and mauve are better for a mature, unobtrusive, natural look.

- ☐ Pink and lilac eye shadow can make eyes look tired and sore, so use with care and other colours.

- ☐ Dark eye shadow can also be used as eyeliner on fairer skins.

Remember, as always, that light draws forward and dark takes back.

Contraindications

The usual contraindications to skin care product apply to using eye shadow, but add to these, watery or sensitive eyes.

Applying eye shadow

- ☐ Make sure your client's eyes are closed and not directly facing a bright light.

- ☐ Hold tissue underneath lower lashes to catch any excess eye shadow and avoid staining of the base make-up.

- ☐ All eye shadows must be selected in advance and scraped onto a palette. To avoid cross-infection, eye shadow must NEVER be applied directly from the container.

- ☐ Apply using sanitised or disposable brushes or foam-tipped applicator.

- ☐ Apply colour remembering that light colours highlight and attract darker colours detract and create shadow.

- ☐ Always complete both eyes simultaneously, i.e. whatever you apply to one eye you should immediately replicate on the other in order to achieve balance.

- ☐ Blend with fingers or brushes over middle and outer part of the lid towards the eyebrow arch, leaving no hard line.

- ☐ Keep checking that colour is balanced on both eyes. By asking the client to open their eyes at regular stages of the eye make-up application.

Eyeliner

Eyeliner is used to define the shape of the eye. Harder lines are used for fashionable effects, while softer lines are preferable for natural looks and more mature clients. You can choose eye liner colour to:

- match the mascara, or
- match the eye colour, or
- match or accentuate the eye shadow.

Eyeliner comes in several forms.

- **Liquid** – gum or oil based in water; applied with a soft brush or tipped applicator
- **Cakes or blocks of water colour powder** – this is now used less often, but may be wetted or applied with a damp brush, and the water content varied to create a harder or softer line.
- **Crayon or pencil** – wax or oil stick; can be blended like eye shadow or sharpened to produce a hard line
- **Kohl (kajal)** – soft, black, wax pencil; applied to inner rims of the eye and/or the eyelid.

Contraindications

The usual contraindications to using skin care products apply (see Topic 3 above), but add to these, contact lenses and/or sore eyes. It is also advisable not to use eyeliner below the eyes if the skin is crepey.

Applying eyeliner

- Use sanitised or disposable brushes or sharpened pencils.
- Ask your client to close her eyes when applying eyeliner to upper lids, and to look away from the applicator when applying it to the lower lids.
- Keep your hand steady – you can rest it gently on a tissue on your client's face if necessary.
- Do not press down on the eye.
- Do not lean on the client.
- Lift the skin from below the brow, to place the line as close to the lashes as possible (unless you are drawing above the lash line to give an enlarging effect).
- Apply eyeliner from the centre to the outer edges.
- Soften the line with a sponge or cotton bud if preferred.
- Check that thickness and shaper are balanced on both eyes.

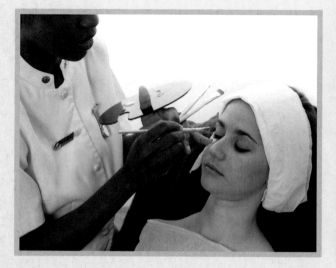
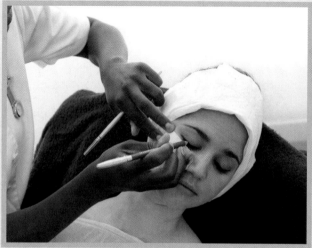

Mascara

Mascara is used to thicken, colour and lengthen eyelashes to enhance the shape and colour of the eyes. It comes in various colours to match the darkest colours of the eye shadow or eyeliner used, or to match false eyelashes or, for a natural look, to complement hair colour. Ideally, it should also be:

☐ long lasting

☐ run proof

☐ hypoallergenic

☐ easy to apply.

There are several types of mascara.

☐ **Block/cake** – this is pigmented and wax based. It is applied with a flat, wet brush, but its use is becoming less common.

☐ **Cream** – easy to apply and remove, but not run proof or waterproof, so rarely used in salons.

☐ **Liquid** – resin based with pigments in water (or alcohol and water) with oil to soften; use with a disposable brush; can have special lash-building features; generally easy to remove.

Contraindications

In addition to general contraindications and those that specifically apply to products used in the eye area, see Topic 3 above, mascara is contraindicated for the lower lashes if the skin below the eyes is flaky or crepey. In addition, do not use alcohol-based mascara or mascara with filaments on clients who use contact lenses.

Applying mascara

☐ Use disposable spiral brushes or a disinfected flat brush (for block mascara).

☐ Ask your client to look down and relax the upper eyelids when applying mascara to upper lashes, and to look up and away from the brush when applying mascara to lower lashes.

☐ Lift the skin of the eyelids from below the brow, to prevent mascara marking eye make-up.

☐ Apply mascara first downwards over the upper lashes, then upwards underneath the lashes to make sure every part is covered.

☐ Place a tissue under the lower lashes to protect the skin.

☐ Build up the mascara in fine layers, allowing an interval for each to dry in between, to prevent clogging.

☐ If required, separate lashes afterwards with a lash or brow comb.

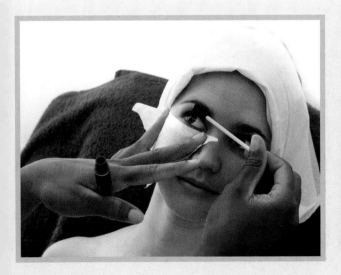
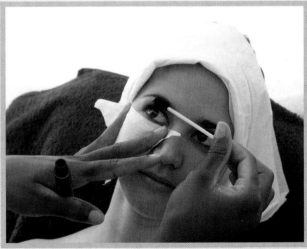

Blusher

As well as contouring, blusher colours are used to:

- balance with the eye and lip make-up
- give the face a healthy glow
- even out skin tones.

In general, use:

- pastel colours to soften features
- bright colours to accentuate features and add warmth
- dark colours to recede features
- matt colours for daytime and iridescent for eveningwear.

As colours can look quite different when applied over different skin colours and foundations, it is good to practise and discover for yourself the different effects when applying cool or warm colours over different coloured skins and in conjunction with other make-up colours. Remind yourself of some of the characteristics of skin colouring to bear in mind when using make-up products that we looked at in Topic 3. You could build up your own colour chart with notes on the effects you have produced.

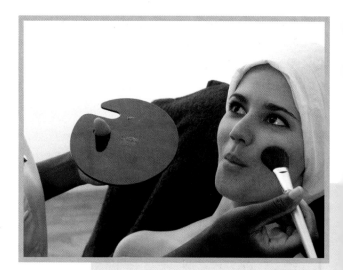

Applying blushers

- Use very soft, round-ended brushes to apply and blend in powders. Tap off any excess from the brush before applying.
- Use small sponges or fingers to apply liquid or cream blushers.
- Blend blushers upwards and outwards.
- Do not apply blusher too near the eyes or nose. Start the blusher on the cheekbones directly below the centre line of the eye and do not drop below the level of the corner of the nose, otherwise the facial contours will appear to be dragged downwards.
- Check that you are applying the cosmetics in a balanced way on both sides of the face.
- Use stronger contouring for evening, photographic and fashion wear.

Lip liner

Lip liners are wax-based pencils used to contour lips to the desired shape (see Topic 3) and to stop lipstick 'bleeding' into other make-up and into the lines around the mouth.

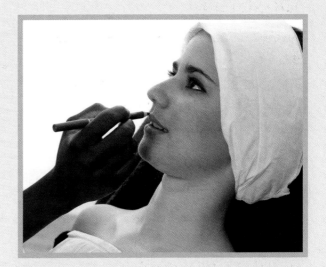

Applying lip liner

☐ Apply after foundation, powder, eye make-up, blusher, shader or highlighter, but before lipstick.

☐ Always sharpen the pencil to obtain a clean surface and fine line.

Contraindications are the same as those for lipstick.

Lipstick

Lipsticks, in addition to being a shaping tool (see Topic 3) are designed to:

☐ add balance and colour

☐ enhance the lips

☐ express style or personality and give a finished look to 'smart' presentation

☐ protect the lips from sun, cold and wind.

Lipsticks come in various forms.

☐ **Conventional sticks** – wax based with softeners, such as lanolin, mineral oils or petroleum jelly; provide excellent coverage; can be pearlised, matte, gloss and with lip balm or sun-block protection.

☐ **Tubes** – for glossy or creamy finish.

☐ **Pots** – add sheer (transparent) colour to lips, giving a more natural look.

Lipstick colours

Lipstick colours should balance with make-up and clothing colours.

☐ Strong colours balance well with muted eye make-up and draw attention to lips.

☐ Deeper colours are needed if redefining new lip shapes, especially around the edges of the new lines.

☐ Pale, glossy or pearlised lipsticks give a fuller effect to lips, while deeper colours reduce the appearance of fullness.

Contraindications

As well as general contraindications and those for make-up products, excessively dry or cracked lips are contraindicated for lip liner and lipstick.

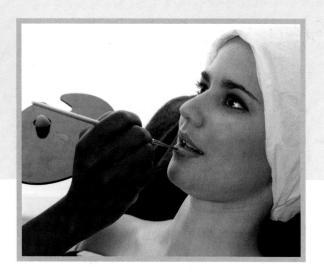

Applying lipstick

☐ To avoid cross-infection, never apply using the stick itself. Always scrape the required amount onto a palette and then use a disinfected or disposable lip brush to apply.

☐ Fill in lipstick after foundation, powder (if used) and lip liner.

☐ Protect surrounding make-up with a tissue.

☐ Use a tissue to blot and fix the first application of lipstick by brushing a layer of powder over the tissue.

☐ Repeat as above.

Lip gloss

Lip gloss is a clear or coloured gel available in a pot or stick form. It can be applied on its own (as for lipstick, see above) or over lipstick to give a gloss effect. It creates the illusion of fuller lips, is often used for glamour or evening wear and is easy to remove.

Order of application of make-up

Products should be applied in the following sequence, unless otherwise indicated above:

1. Pre-base
2. Corrective creams
3. Foundation
4. Concealer
5. Powder
6. Shader
7. Highlighter
8. Eye shadow
9. Eyeliner
10. Mascara
11. Blusher
12. Lip liner
13. Lipstick
14. Lip gloss (where appropriate)
15. Show the make-up to the client

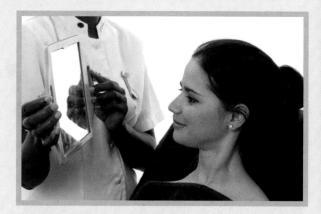

> ### KEY POINT
> All make-up products should be decanted onto a palette before application with a sterilised or disposable applicator, such as a brush or sponge. This will help reduce cross infection.

Acceptable time limits

The time limit acceptable to the industry for a cleanse and day make-up is up to 30 minutes.

However, if the client requested a special make-up, e.g. for a wedding or evening it could take up to an hour. If a client required a make-up lesson, an hour would be required to ensure enough time was allocated for the client to learn the routine and appropriate application on themselves.

Client record card

For more information on the record card see Chapter 1. It is essential to consult and fill in the client record card at every visit.

Changes in the skin analysis and treatment plan should be recorded, as well as notes on all the products used (colours and makes) and any reactions to these. Your notes can then be used for future reference by yourself or another therapist.

Sterilisation and sanitisation of make-up tools

See Chapter 1 for information on sterilisation methods for therapy tools. The key points to remember for make-up tools are:

- [ ] always use cleaned and sterilised brushes and sponges
- [ ] soak sponges in sterilising solution for at least an hour, then rinse thoroughly in clean water
- [ ] after cleaning brushes thoroughly in hot, soapy water, wipe them with alcohol or sanitiser before allowing them to dry
- [ ] allow sponges and brushes to dry naturally and thoroughly
- [ ] put them in a sanitising unit until they are next used
- [ ] Thoroughly scrub clean and disinfect make-up palettes between uses
- [ ] never use broken or cracked containers as they can store germs.

Alternatively, you could use disposable applicators and/or palettes.

ENDPOINTS

After this section, you should understand:

- [ ] how to prepare client and working area for a make-up session
- [ ] the capabilities, uses and application of a range of make-up products
- [ ] the order of application for make-up
- [ ] acceptable time-limits for a make-up treatment
- [ ] the sterilisation and sanitisation of make-up tools
- [ ] the requirements of good record-keeping.

Chapter 5:
Manicure and pedicure

In this chapter we'll be looking at:

Topic 1:
The structure of the lower limbs, feet and hands

Topic 2:
The structure and function of the nail

Topic 3:
Nail conditions, diseases and disorders

Topic 4:
Preparations for manicures and pedicures

Topic 5:
Nail shapes, massage and manicure treatments

Topic 6:
Specialised treatments and nail enhancements

Topic 7:
Pedicure treatments

introduction

The main purpose of manicures and pedicures is to keep nails, hands and feet in good condition. We have covered the structure of the skin, skeletal, muscular and circulatory systems of the hands and feet in previous chapters.

Topic 1: The structure of the lower limbs, feet and hands

We looked at the general structure, nature and diseases of the skeletal, muscular and circulatory systems of the body in Chapter 2. Here we will summarise the points that are specific to the lower limbs, feet and hands.

The skeleton of the lower limbs, feet and hands

The bones of the lower limbs, feet and hands form part of the appendicular skeleton. The appendicular skeleton is made up of the shoulder and pelvic girdles, arms and legs. The bones that make up the parts of the appendicular skeleton include:

Shoulder girdle: two scapulae and two clavicles

Arm: one humerus, one ulna, one radius
(each arm)

Wrist: eight carpal bones (each wrist)

Hand: five metacarpal bones (each palm of hand)

Fingers: 14 phalanges in each hand, two in the thumb and three each in the fingers

Pelvic girdle: two innominate bones
(each one including an ilium, ischium and pubis)

Leg: one femur, one tibia, one fibula and one patella (each leg)

Ankle: seven tarsals (each foot)

Foot: five metatarsals (each foot)

Toes: 14 phalanges in each foot, two in each big toe and three in each of the other toes.

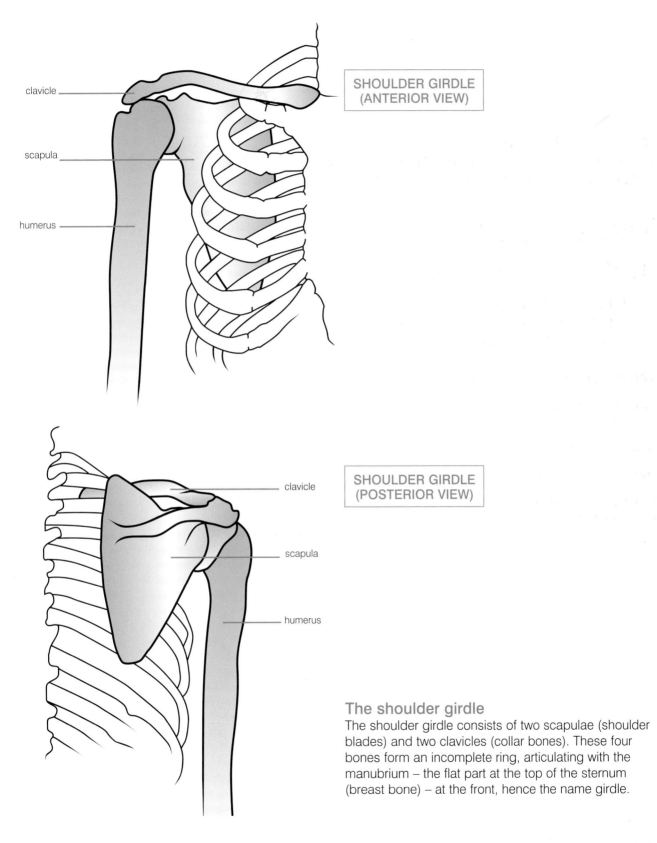

SHOULDER GIRDLE
(ANTERIOR VIEW)

clavicle

scapula

humerus

SHOULDER GIRDLE
(POSTERIOR VIEW)

clavicle

scapula

humerus

The shoulder girdle

The shoulder girdle consists of two scapulae (shoulder blades) and two clavicles (collar bones). These four bones form an incomplete ring, articulating with the manubrium – the flat part at the top of the sternum (breast bone) – at the front, hence the name girdle.

The pelvic girdle

The pelvic girdle is formed by two large innominate bones which meet in front at the symphysis pubis and articulate with the sacrum in the back to form a ring of bone.

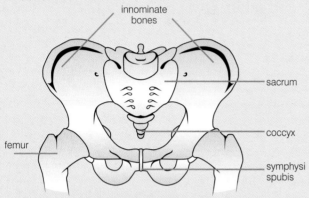

THE PELVIC GIRDLE (ANTERIOR VIEW)

The innominate bones, with the sacrum and coccyx, form the pelvis which surrounds the pelvic cavity. The pelvis of the female is wider and shallower than that of the male. Each innominate bone is formed by the fusion of three parts – an ilium, an ischium and a pubis. At the junction of these is a socket for the head of the femur.

The arm and hand

Arms and legs have the same basic layout of bones within them but different names are given to them. The bones of the upper limb and hand are the:

Carpals (wrist bones): eight in each wrist arranged in two rows of four: upper row (nearest arm) are called the scaphoid, lunate, triquetral and pisiform; the lower row (joining the metacarpal bones) are called the trapezium, the trapezoid, the capitate and the hamate.

Metacarpals (palm bones): five in each hand.

Phalanges (finger bones): 14 in each hand; two in each thumb and three in each of the other fingers

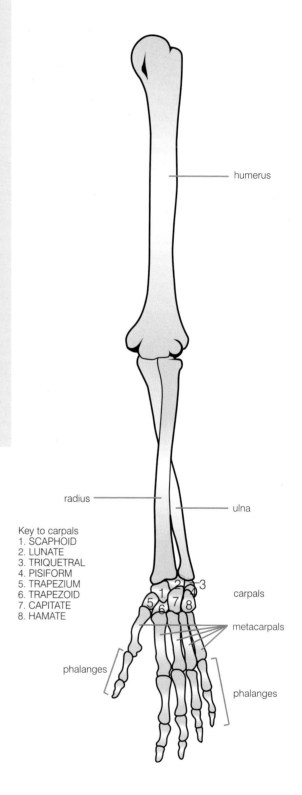

Key to carpals
1. SCAPHOID
2. LUNATE
3. TRIQUETRAL
4. PISIFORM
5. TRAPEZIUM
6. TRAPEZOID
7. CAPITATE
8. HAMATE

The leg and foot

The bones of the leg and foot include the:

Tarsals: seven in each ankle/heel: the talus joins the foot to the leg and is a principal part of the ankle joint, the calcaneus (the heel bone) projects backwards; the navicular bone lies between the talus and cuneiform bones, there are three wedge-shaped cuneiform bones, the medial, intermediate and lateral and finally the cuboid bone on the lateral side of the foot, which is between the calcaneus and the metatarsals.

Metatarsals: five in each foot.

Phalanges: 14 in each foot, two in each big toe and three in each of the other toes.

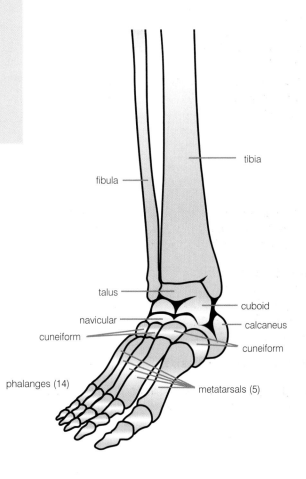

The principal muscles of the lower limbs, feet and hands

There are hundreds of muscles in the body. The diagrams in this section show the principal muscles of the lower limbs, feet and hands, detailing their position and their action.

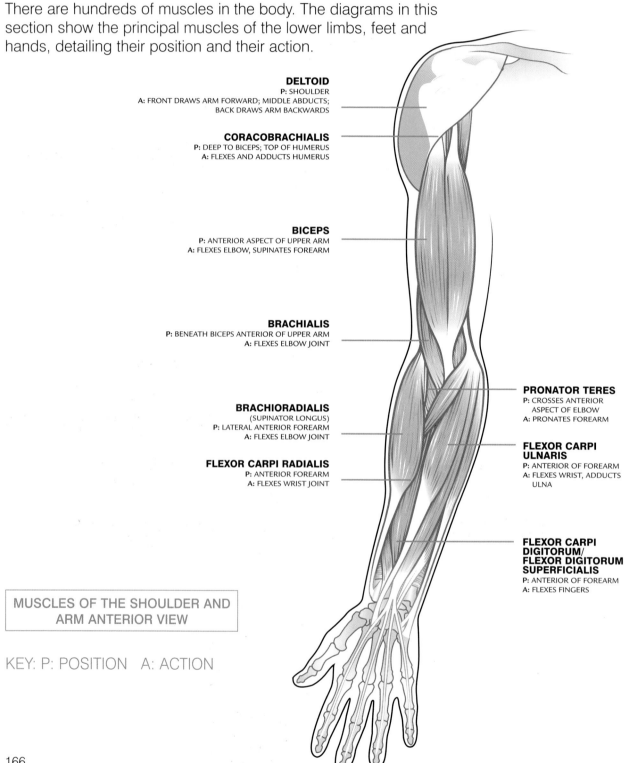

DELTOID
P: SHOULDER
A: FRONT DRAWS ARM FORWARD; MIDDLE ABDUCTS; BACK DRAWS ARM BACKWARDS

CORACOBRACHIALIS
P: DEEP TO BICEPS; TOP OF HUMERUS
A: FLEXES AND ADDUCTS HUMERUS

BICEPS
P: ANTERIOR ASPECT OF UPPER ARM
A: FLEXES ELBOW, SUPINATES FOREARM

BRACHIALIS
P: BENEATH BICEPS ANTERIOR OF UPPER ARM
A: FLEXES ELBOW JOINT

BRACHIORADIALIS
(SUPINATOR LONGUS)
P: LATERAL ANTERIOR FOREARM
A: FLEXES ELBOW JOINT

FLEXOR CARPI RADIALIS
P: ANTERIOR FOREARM
A: FLEXES WRIST JOINT

PRONATOR TERES
P: CROSSES ANTERIOR ASPECT OF ELBOW
A: PRONATES FOREARM

FLEXOR CARPI ULNARIS
P: ANTERIOR OF FOREARM
A: FLEXES WRIST, ADDUCTS ULNA

FLEXOR CARPI DIGITORUM/ FLEXOR DIGITORUM SUPERFICIALIS
P: ANTERIOR OF FOREARM
A: FLEXES FINGERS

MUSCLES OF THE SHOULDER AND ARM ANTERIOR VIEW

KEY: P: POSITION   A: ACTION

166

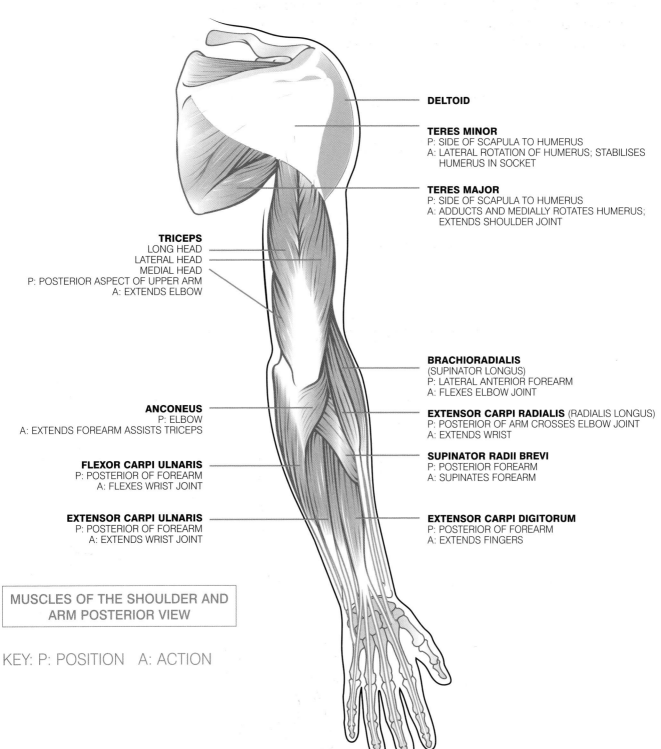

DELTOID

TERES MINOR
P: SIDE OF SCAPULA TO HUMERUS
A: LATERAL ROTATION OF HUMERUS; STABILISES
HUMERUS IN SOCKET

TERES MAJOR
P: SIDE OF SCAPULA TO HUMERUS
A: ADDUCTS AND MEDIALLY ROTATES HUMERUS;
EXTENDS SHOULDER JOINT

TRICEPS
LONG HEAD
LATERAL HEAD
MEDIAL HEAD
P: POSTERIOR ASPECT OF UPPER ARM
A: EXTENDS ELBOW

BRACHIORADIALIS
(SUPINATOR LONGUS)
P: LATERAL ANTERIOR FOREARM
A: FLEXES ELBOW JOINT

ANCONEUS
P: ELBOW
A: EXTENDS FOREARM ASSISTS TRICEPS

EXTENSOR CARPI RADIALIS (RADIALIS LONGUS)
P: POSTERIOR OF ARM CROSSES ELBOW JOINT
A: EXTENDS WRIST

SUPINATOR RADII BREVI
P: POSTERIOR FOREARM
A: SUPINATES FOREARM

FLEXOR CARPI ULNARIS
P: POSTERIOR OF FOREARM
A: FLEXES WRIST JOINT

EXTENSOR CARPI ULNARIS
P: POSTERIOR OF FOREARM
A: EXTENDS WRIST JOINT

EXTENSOR CARPI DIGITORUM
P: POSTERIOR OF FOREARM
A: EXTENDS FINGERS

MUSCLES OF THE SHOULDER AND
ARM POSTERIOR VIEW

KEY: P: POSITION   A: ACTION

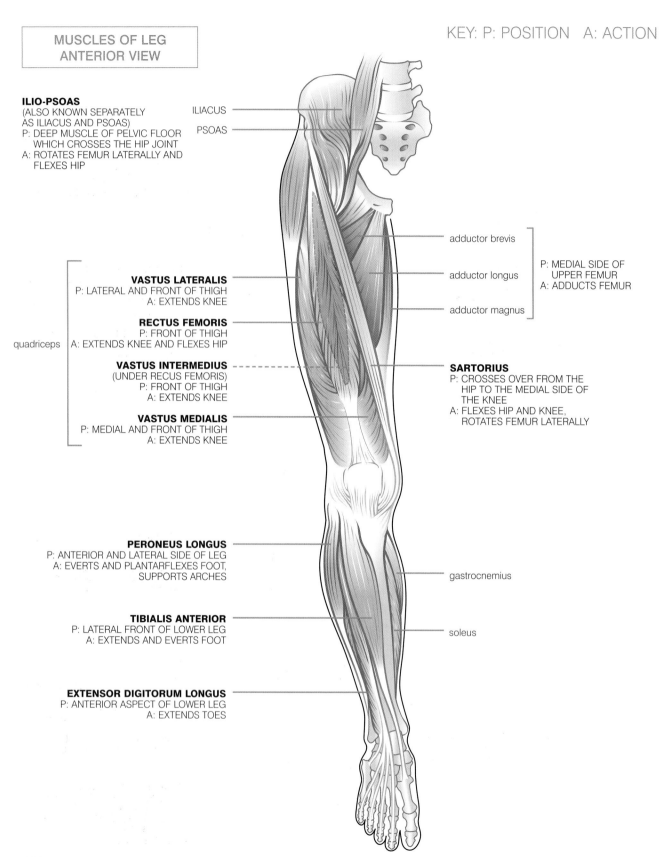

KEY: P: POSITION   A: ACTION

MUSCLES OF LEG
ANTERIOR VIEW

ILIO-PSOAS
(ALSO KNOWN SEPARATELY
AS ILIACUS AND PSOAS)
P: DEEP MUSCLE OF PELVIC FLOOR
   WHICH CROSSES THE HIP JOINT
A: ROTATES FEMUR LATERALLY AND
   FLEXES HIP

ILIACUS

PSOAS

adductor brevis

adductor longus

P: MEDIAL SIDE OF
   UPPER FEMUR
A: ADDUCTS FEMUR

adductor magnus

VASTUS LATERALIS
P: LATERAL AND FRONT OF THIGH
A: EXTENDS KNEE

RECTUS FEMORIS
P: FRONT OF THIGH
A: EXTENDS KNEE AND FLEXES HIP

quadriceps

VASTUS INTERMEDIUS
(UNDER RECUS FEMORIS)
P: FRONT OF THIGH
A: EXTENDS KNEE

SARTORIUS
P: CROSSES OVER FROM THE
   HIP TO THE MEDIAL SIDE OF
   THE KNEE
A: FLEXES HIP AND KNEE,
   ROTATES FEMUR LATERALLY

VASTUS MEDIALIS
P: MEDIAL AND FRONT OF THIGH
A: EXTENDS KNEE

PERONEUS LONGUS
P: ANTERIOR AND LATERAL SIDE OF LEG
A: EVERTS AND PLANTARFLEXES FOOT,
   SUPPORTS ARCHES

gastrocnemius

TIBIALIS ANTERIOR
P: LATERAL FRONT OF LOWER LEG
A: EXTENDS AND EVERTS FOOT

soleus

EXTENSOR DIGITORUM LONGUS
P: ANTERIOR ASPECT OF LOWER LEG
A: EXTENDS TOES

KEY: P: POSITION   A: ACTION

MUSCLES OF THE LEG
POSTERIOR VIEW

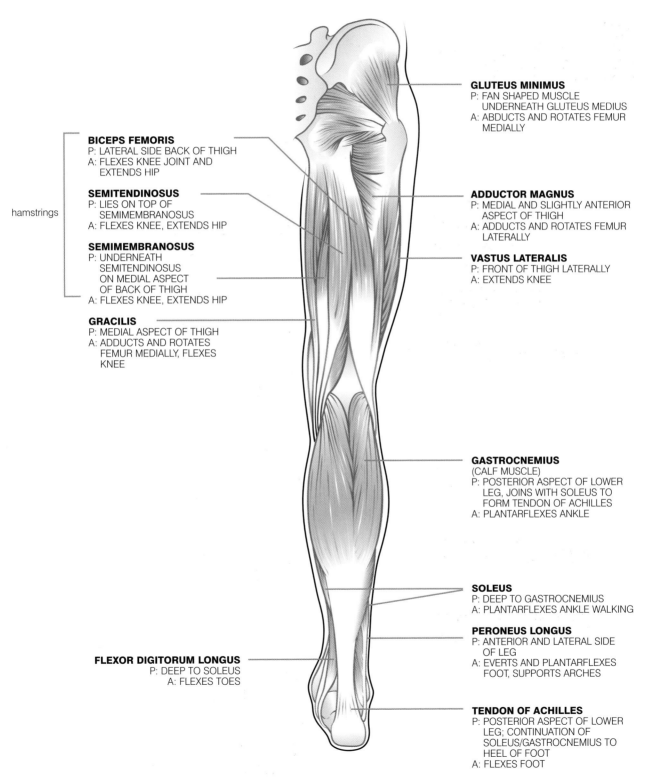

BICEPS FEMORIS
P: LATERAL SIDE BACK OF THIGH
A: FLEXES KNEE JOINT AND
   EXTENDS HIP

SEMITENDINOSUS
P: LIES ON TOP OF
   SEMIMEMBRANOSUS
A: FLEXES KNEE, EXTENDS HIP

hamstrings

SEMIMEMBRANOSUS
P: UNDERNEATH
   SEMITENDINOSUS
   ON MEDIAL ASPECT
   OF BACK OF THIGH
A: FLEXES KNEE, EXTENDS HIP

GRACILIS
P: MEDIAL ASPECT OF THIGH
A: ADDUCTS AND ROTATES
   FEMUR MEDIALLY, FLEXES
   KNEE

GLUTEUS MINIMUS
P: FAN SHAPED MUSCLE
   UNDERNEATH GLUTEUS MEDIUS
A: ABDUCTS AND ROTATES FEMUR
   MEDIALLY

ADDUCTOR MAGNUS
P: MEDIAL AND SLIGHTLY ANTERIOR
   ASPECT OF THIGH
A: ADDUCTS AND ROTATES FEMUR
   LATERALLY

VASTUS LATERALIS
P: FRONT OF THIGH LATERALLY
A: EXTENDS KNEE

GASTROCNEMIUS
(CALF MUSCLE)
P: POSTERIOR ASPECT OF LOWER
   LEG, JOINS WITH SOLEUS TO
   FORM TENDON OF ACHILLES
A: PLANTARFLEXES ANKLE

SOLEUS
P: DEEP TO GASTROCNEMIUS
A: PLANTARFLEXES ANKLE WALKING

PERONEUS LONGUS
P: ANTERIOR AND LATERAL SIDE
   OF LEG
A: EVERTS AND PLANTARFLEXES
   FOOT, SUPPORTS ARCHES

FLEXOR DIGITORUM LONGUS
P: DEEP TO SOLEUS
A: FLEXES TOES

TENDON OF ACHILLES
P: POSTERIOR ASPECT OF LOWER
   LEG; CONTINUATION OF
   SOLEUS/GASTROCNEMIUS TO
   HEEL OF FOOT
A: FLEXES FOOT

169

The main arteries and veins of the lower limbs, feet and hands

The following diagrams show the main veins and arteries that feed the lower limbs, feet and hands.

ARM MAIN ARTERIES

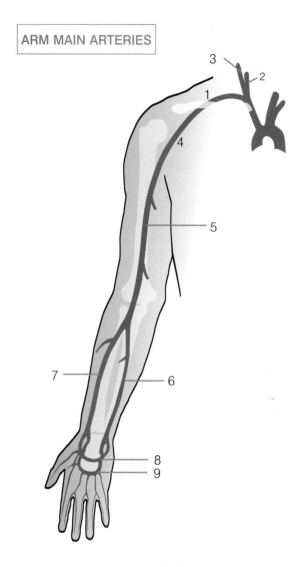

ARM MAIN VEINS

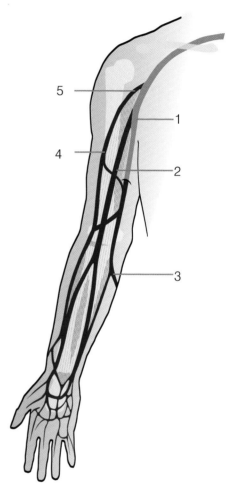

1. right subclavian
2. right common carotid
3. vertebral
4. axillary
5. brachial
6. right ulnar
7. right radial
8. right deep palmar arch
9. right superficial palmar arch

1. right axillary
2. right brachial
3. right basilic
4. right cephalic
5. right subclavian

LEG MAIN ARTERIES

LEG MAIN VEINS

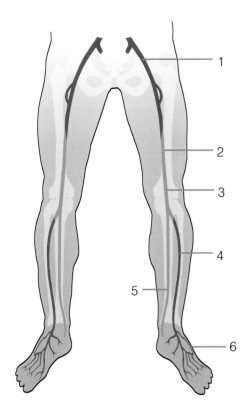

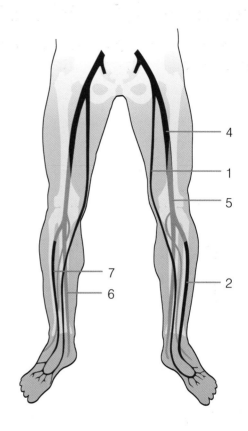

1. external iliac
2. left femoral
3. left popliteal
4. left anterior tibial
5. left posterior tibial
6. plantar arch

1. long saphenous
2. left short saphenous
3. dorsal venous arch
4. left femoral
5. left popliteal
6. right posterior tibial
7. right anterior tibial

ENDPOINTS
At the end of this topic, you should know the

☐ position of the main components of the appendicular skeleton

☐ position of the main arteries and veins in the lower limbs, feet and hands

☐ position of the main muscles in the lower limbs, feet and hands.

Topic 2: The structure and function of the nail

The fingernail, or nail plate, serves to protect the end of the fingertip and to enhance the sensitivity of the nerves in the fingertip. The nail we see is itself a plate of translucent keratin, but it is part of a system that continually replenishes the nail plate, and protects and seals the system from infection and the environment.

The components of the nail system

The nail system that lies beneath the nail has six main components, each with a specific purpose, and each shown in the diagrams below. These are the:

- free edge
- hyponychium
- peronychium (lateral nail fold)
- eponychium (cuticle)
- nail plate
- cuticle
- nail bed
- nail folds
- matrix
- mantle
- lunula
- nail wall

Free edge
The free edge of the nail is the part extending beyond the end of the skin of the fingertip.

Hyponychium
The hyponychium forms a seal between the free edge of the nail and the skin of the fingertip.

Peronychium
The paronychial edge or peronichium is the skin that overlaps the sides of the nail. The peronichium is the site of paronicia infections, hangnails and ingrowing nails.

Eponychium
The eponychium forms a seal between the skin and the nail plate that protects the underlying matrix from infection.

Nail plate
What we commonly call the fingernail is actually the nail plate, a protective shield of translucent keratin for the nail bed beneath. Grooves in the underneath of the plate help to hold it to the nail bed. While the nail plate is actually translucent, the blood vessels beneath it give it a pink appearance.

Cuticle
It protects the matrix from infection.

Nail bed
As the matrix produces new cells, pushing the nail forward, the nail moves along the nail bed, which adds cells to the underside of the nail, thickening and strengthening it as it grows. The nail bed contains the

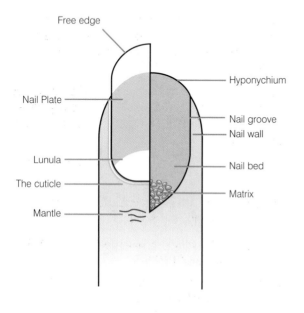

THE STRUCTURE OF THE NAIL

Free edge
Hyponychium
Nail Plate
Nail groove
Nail wall
Lunula
Nail bed
The cuticle
Matrix
Mantle

blood vessels (which, seen through the translucent nail plate, give the nail its colour), the nerves that provide sensation and melanocytes. The nail bed lies directly beneath the nail plate. Both have grooves which dovetail into each other, holding the nail plate in place as it grows forward.

Nail folds

The nail folds are the folds in the skin which protect the matrix, and in which the edges of the nail plate sit. The root of the nail is protected by the proximal nail fold, and the edges by the lateral nail folds.

Matrix

The matrix is where the cells of the nail plate and nail bed are produced. It lies mostly beneath the nail and the nail bed with only the tip of the root visible through the nail plate as the lunula. The matrix produces keratin cells for the nail plate and bed, pushing older cells forward along the finger or toe as it does so.

Mantle

Deep fold of skin at the base of the nail before the cuticle.

Lunula

The half moon on our fingernails, or lunula, is actually the visible front end of the germinal matrix extending underneath the nail plate. The prominence of the lunula varies from person to person, and is normally most visible on the thumbnails. The shape of the lunula is reflected in the natural shape of the free edge of the nail.

Nail wall

The folds of skin which overlap the sides of the nail plate for protection.

How the nail grows

Nail growth rate varies, but may be up to 3 mm per week for fingernails and 1 mm for toenails, with the whole fingernail being replaced two or three times per year, and the toenail every year to 18 months. The growth rate peaks in our early teens and then reduces with age, but it may increase again during pregnancy, the summer, or while we sleep.

Factors affecting nail growth

Nail growth and health can be affected by a range of factors, including:

☐ **Health** – the shape, integrity and colour of the nail can be affected by diseases of the lung, heart, kidney, liver or thyroid.

☐ **Age** – the growth rate of both fingernails and toenails slows as we get older, and the protein in the nail becomes more brittle and prone to splitting.

☐ **Diet** – while serious vitamin or mineral deficiencies may affect the nails, diet does not generally cause abnormal nail changes, except in cases of severe malnutrition.

☐ **Medication** – medication may affect the rate at which fast-growing cells in the body reproduce

☐ **Climate** – blood increases in hotter climates thereby increasing nail growth.

☐ **Damage** – if the matrix is damaged nail growth can be affected or retarded.

☐ **Lifestyle** – environmental factors, eg hands in water, or chemical solutions.

ENDPOINTS

You should now understand:

☐ the components of the nail system

☐ how the nail grows.

Topic 3: Nail conditions, diseases and disorders

There are many specific nail conditions, some of which are localised to the nails, while others may be related to more general medical conditions. You need to be able to recognise them and to know which ones are contraindicated for treatments.

Finding out about nail conditions

Nail conditions are not always immediately obvious. Your starting points to finding out about your client's nails are:

☐ your client's consultation card (if your client has been before)

☐ communicating with your client

☐ preliminary visual check and initial cleanse.

If you have treated the client before, check the client's record card for any existing conditions and previous treatments before your client arrives. The record card must be updated on each visit, with any new observations, as existing conditions can change and new ones arise.

Wipe the hands with sanitiser, and remove any enamel before checking for contraindications.

Salon Name
Client Consultation Form – *Manicure and Pedicure Treatments*

Client Name: Date:
Address:

                                                     Profession:
e-mail: Tel. No: Day
                                                              Eve

PERSONAL DETAILS:
Age group: Under 20☐ 20–30☐ 30–40☐ 40–50☐ 50–60☐ 60+☐
Lifestyle: Active☐ Sedentary☐
Last visit to the doctor:
GP Address:
No. of children (if applicable):
Date of last period (if applicable):

DISEASES AND DISORDERS *(select where/if appropriate)*:

Transverse ridges ☐	Leuconychia ☐	Onychatrophia ☐
Vertical ridges ☐	Flaking ☐	Onychauxis ☐
Beau's lines ☐	Onychorrhexis ☐	Onychgryposis ☐
Blue nails ☐	Pitting ☐	Onychocryptosis ☐
Psoriasis ☐	Pterygium ☐	Koilonychia ☐
Tinea Ungium ☐	Onychia ☐	Onychophagy ☐
Tinea Pedis ☐	Hang nail ☐	Koilonychia ☐
Paronychia (Whitlow) ☐	Lamella dystrophy ☐	Warts ☐
Sepsis ☐	Onychomycosis ☐	

CONTRAINDICATIONS REQUIRING MEDICAL PERMISSION – in circumstances where medical permission cannot be obtained clients must give their informed consent in writing prior to treatment *(select if/where appropriate)*:

Haemophilia ☐	Recent operations affecting the area ☐
Any condition being treated by a GP, dermatologist or another practitioner ☐	Diabetes ☐
	Inflamed nerve ☐
Acute Arthritis ☐	Undiagnosed pain ☐
Medical oedema ☐	Acute rheumatism ☐
Nervous/Psychotic conditions ☐	

CONTRAINDICATIONS THAT RESTRICT TREATMENT *(select where/if appropriate)*:

Fever ☐	Recent fractures (minimum 3 months) ☐
Contagious or infectious diseases ☐	Sunburn ☐
Diarrhoea and vomiting ☐	Repetitive strain injury ☐
Under the influence of recreational drugs or alcohol ☐	Carpal Tunnel Syndrome ☐
	Severely bitten or damaged nails ☐
Any known allergies ☐	Nail separation ☐
Undiagnosed lumps and bumps ☐	Eczema ☐
Inflammation ☐	Psoriasis ☐
Cuts ☐	Verucca ☐
Severe bruising ☐	Loss of skin sensation ☐
Abrasions ☐	Chilblains ☐
Scar tissue (2 years for major operation and 6 months for a small scar) ☐	Corns ☐

NAIL TEST *(select where/if appropriate)*:

Moisture content:	Excellent ☐	Good ☐	Fair ☐	Poor ☐
Cuticle condition:	Excellent ☐	Good ☐	Fair ☐	Poor ☐
Skin condition:	Dehydrated ☐	Dry ☐	Normal ☐	
Skins healing ability:	Excellent ☐	Good ☐	Fair ☐	Poor ☐
Circulation:	Good ☐	Normal ☐	Poor ☐	

What to look out for

Onychosis is the technical term for a nail disease. Pronounce the 'onych' part of the technical terms 'on-eek'. It comes from the Greek for nail or claw.

Ridges and furrows

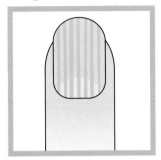

Superficial ridges (corrugations) – possibly the result of age (with thickening of nails) or illness

Longitudinal (vertical ridges) – possibly associated with ill health

Single ridges – result of trauma, constant picking or ill health

Single transverse (horizontal) furrow (Beau's lines) – possibly the result of ill health.

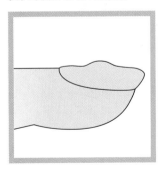

Deep furrows – possibly the result of dermatitis (see below) or ill health

Ridges and furrows can generally be buffed to make them smoother.

Pitting

Pitting is a sign of an underlying problem, such as dermatitis or psoriasis (see below), which can be a contraindication; if severe, suggest that your client seeks medical attention.

White spots (leuconychia)

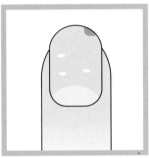

This is a common condition generally caused by an injury to the nail matrix, allowing an air pocket to form. The nails can be treated gently to avoid further injury.

Brittle nails (onychorrhexis)

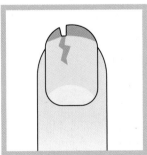

Poor blood supply, caused by anaemia, illness or use of over-strong detergents removing natural oils, has dried the nails making them brittle, with a tendency to break easily. Regular use of cuticle cream, manicures, moisturiser and good diet should help this condition.

Hang nail

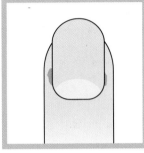

The cuticle has split as it has adhered to the nail plate and cannot continue to move forward with the growth of the nail, causing the cuticle to split leaving it prone to infection. Cut the torn cuticle carefully with cuticle clippers, and soften with cuticle cream/oil. Suggest regular manicures to the client as these will help prevent recurrence.

Discoloured nails

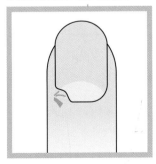

Blue nail – may be caused by poor circulation, anaemia or a heart problem. Using massage cream and finger exercises should help circulation.

Black nail – usually the result of heavy bruising. If particularly severe, the nail plate may detach from the nail bed, but a new nail usually grows to replace it. Treat very gently, avoiding pressure. If severe, avoid the nail until a new nail is in place.

Stained – nails can be stained by several things, including nicotine, dark nail enamels and hair dyes. Advise your client about the possible cause of the staining and buff nails regularly to reduce stains and encourage new nail growth.
Discolouration due to ringworm – see below.

Flaking (lamella dystrophy)

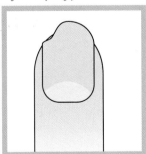

Flaking can be due to biting, incorrect or severe hand and nail treatments, lengthy exposure to hot

water or harsh chemicals, or to general ill health. Keeping the nails short, moisturising and regular manicure with home-care advice should cure this condition.

Overgrowth of the cuticle (pterygium)

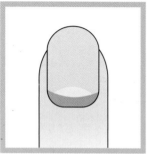

The cuticle has a hardened growth which has grown over and stuck to the nail plate. Treat by softening the cuticle with oil or paraffin wax, then gently pushing it back and removing the excess cuticle carefully with nail clippers. Regular massage and manicures should prevent the condition recurring.

Excessive thickening (onychauxis or claw nail)

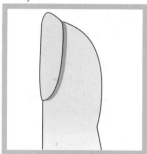

The nail plate has thickened and in some cases discoloured, usually due to internal disorders, infection,

damage below the nail, or to constant rubbing (for instance by a badly fitting shoe). If not infected, the nail may be filed smooth, buffed and shaped as usual. Infections are contraindications to treatment and your client should seek medical advice.

Enlarged nail with increased curve (onychogryphosis)

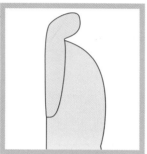

Similar to claw nail; the nail plate has thickened and curved over due to an increase in the horny cells of the nail plate. This is a common complaint in older people, especially if combined with ill-fitting shoes or neglect. It should be treated by a chiropodist or advise medical attention.

Nail is becoming smaller (onychatrophia)

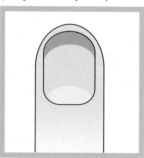

As it becomes smaller, the nail becomes opaque

and ridged and sometimes wastes away completely. It is usually caused by injury under the nail, nervous disorders or disease and manicures are not advised. The nail should be protected from products such as detergents. Advise your client to seek medical advice.

Spoon-shaped nail (koilonychia)

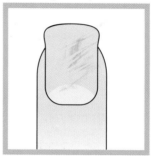

An abnormal growth causes the nail to splay at the sides, with a depression in the middle. It can be hereditary or due to a type of anaemia or overactive thyroid. If possible, the underlying cause should be treated medically.

Ingrowing nails (onychocryptosis)

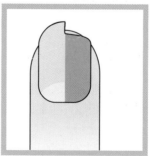

Most often affecting the big toe, the side of the nail plate grows into the flesh of the nail wall.

Ingrowing nails are usually caused by incorrect cutting or filing too far down the sides, ill-fitting shoes or neglect. They can be very painful and inflamed with swelling and pus. If infected, do not treat, advise medical treatment.

Bitten nails (onychophagy)

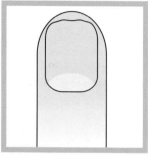

Nail biting reduces the size of the nail so it eventually has no free edge. The nails look ragged and the fingertips sore, increasing chances of infection or hangnails. Regular manicure treatments can help by softening the cuticles, filing the nail edges smooth (if there is enough edge to file) and buffing to encourage growth. However, the condition will only clear up when the biting stops.

Contraindications and infections

In addition to the nail conditions above, some of which may become infectious, there are diseases which are specific to hands, feet and nails which may be contraindicated.

KEY POINT
All infections are contraindicated.

Contraindications requiring medical permission – in circumstances where medical permission cannot be obtained clients must give their informed consent in writing prior to the treatment

☐ Haemophilia	☐ Arthritis	☐ Inflamed nerve
☐ Any condition already being treated by a GP, dermatologist or another practitioner	☐ Nervous/Psychotic conditions	☐ Undiagnosed pain
	☐ Recent operations of the hands or feet	☐ Acute rheumatism
☐ Medical oedema	☐ Diabetes	

Contraindications that restrict treatment

☐ Any form of infection, disease or fever	☐ Severe bruising	☐ Severely bitten/damaged nails
☐ Under the influence of recreational drugs or alcohol	☐ Abrasions	☐ Nail separation
	☐ Scar tissues (2 years for major operation and 6 months for a small scar)	☐ Eczema
☐ Diarrhoea and vomiting		☐ Psoriasis
☐ Any known allergies	☐ Recent fractures (minimum 3 months)	☐ Verrucas
☐ Undiagnosed lumps and bumps		☐ Corns
	☐ Sunburn	☐ Chill blains
☐ Inflammation	☐ Repetitive strain injury	☐ Loss of skin sensation
☐ Cuts	☐ Carpal tunnel	

It is important to be able to recognise the different infections that can affect hands and feet:

Onychia
A bacterial or fungal infection usually caused by a damaged cuticle being infected by biting or thumb sucking, frequent use of detergents or immersion in water. It can be very red and sore. Give advice about prevention and seeking medical treatment.

Ringworm and athletes foot (onycho-mycosis/tinea unguium and tinea pedis)
Fungal infections are the most common form of toe and finger nail infection. Highly infectious ringworm first appears as a yellow-brown discolouration at the free edge. This condition is caused by a fungus attacking the nail plate and bed through the free edge but it can spread to the nail root. The nail thickens and becomes furrowed and spongy and sometimes completely detached. Medical advice is essential. Athletes foot (tinea pedis) is another highly contagious form of ringworm, in which the skin between and under the toes becomes swollen, white and waterlogged. It is contraindicated for manicure/pedicure.

Paronychia (Whitlow)
A bacterial infection of the skin around the nail, which becomes swollen, red and inflamed. Usually caused by

broken skin, rough treatment or injury to the cuticle/nail fold, or exposure to unsterile manicure tools or harsh chemicals. A long-term infection may result in the nail becoming deformed. Medical advice should be sought.

Warts and verrucas

Warts are caused by a virus and generally appear on the hands and fingers, especially where there are hangnails. They appear as raised patches, and are sometimes discoloured and rough. A viral wart infection of the nail fold and nail bed is called periungium viral warts.

Verrucas are compressed warts on the feet. Both warts and verrucas are contagious and contraindicated to manicure/pedicure.

Corns

Corns generally appear over the joints in the toes or on the soles of the feet. They have a central core surrounded by thick skin which thickens further when rubbed, putting painful pressure on nerve endings. The client should be referred to a chiropodist for specialised treatment.

Psoriasis

Psoriasis is characterised by small red patches covered in silvery scales. It can affect the skin around and under the nails. It may itch but if rubbed it can start to bleed and then is open to infection. The cause is unknown it can appear at any age and may be inherited or could be triggered by stress or illness. It is not contagious. It is contraindicated if the lesions are open and weeping.

Eczema and dermatitis

Possibly hereditary or due to allergic reactions, the skin appears very dry and red, it may crack and flake and is usually itchy. Clients may be allergic to the lanolin in creams, the resins in nail hardeners and polishes and some ingredients in nail extensions. Take careful notes of any contra-actions.

ENDPOINTS

You should now understand:

☐ nail conditions and how to find out about them

☐ nail contraindications and infections

Topic 4: Preparations for manicures and pedicures

As for all beauty treatments, good preparation is vital for a successful manicure or pedicure. This will include being aware of any contraindications and taking the appropriate course of action. Good communication with your client and use of the record card are essential, as well as excellent preparation and presentation of your equipment.

The basic tools and products used in manicure and pedicure treatments should always be prepared in advance, be laid out professionally and be easily to hand during the treatment. Further treatments, such as hot oil, paraffin wax or thermal mittens, require other tools and products, but these should be prepared when you know which treatment will be needed (see later for these treatments).

Contraindications and contra-actions

See Chapter 1 and Topic 3 of this chapter for contraindications that should be taken into consideration when giving manicures and pedicures. As ever, your communication with your client is vital, both in finding out whether there are contraindications and in being able to advise the best course with sensitivity.

In addition, be vigilant for contra-actions throughout treatments, using products that could cause allergic reactions, such as arachis (peanut oil), perfumed hand lotions, nail enamels (especially dark red) and nail hardeners. Contra-actions could include erythema (redness and irritation of the skin, especially on the eyelids, around the mouth, on the sides of the neck and chest) when the hands have touched the face. These signs do not necessarily appear at the source of the allergy. Good communication with your client at the start of any session will help you find out whether your client is already aware of any allergies. Check and update your client's record card at all times.

Manicure and pedicure tools and their functions

It is essential to know the correct function for each tool.

Tools	Purpose
Emery board	To file and shape nails
Tipped orange wood stick	To push back cuticles and to clean under the free edge
Spatula	To remove creams from containers
Hoof stick – a rubber-tipped orange wood stick	To push back cuticles on fingers and toes
Cuticle knife	To remove cuticle tissue adhering to nail plate
Cuticle nipper	To remove any excess cuticle still adhering to the nail plate, and for hang nails after using the cuticle knife and hoof stick. Never cut the cuticle itself
Buffer	To polish nails, even out ridges, increase circulation and flow of nutrients to the nail
Scissors and nail clippers	To reduce length of nails
Hard skin remover (rasp and/or cream)	To remove hard skin from balls of feet and heels
Nail brush	To clean the nail plate and free edge
Bowls	To hold clean cotton wool, clients' jewellery, warm water for soaking hands
Cotton wool pads	To wipe tools and tip orange wood sticks
Waste bin and facilities for disposal of contaminated waste	To dispose of waste

Manicure and pedicure products

You also need to know about the products used in manicures and pedicures, their ingredients and purpose.

Product	Ingredients	Purpose
Cuticle massage cream/oil	Fats and waxes, eg beeswax, cocoa butter, white soft paraffin	To soften and nourish cuticle, easier to push back
Cuticle remover	Potassium hydroxide, glycerol counters drying effect of hydroxide), oleic acid, water	To remove excess cuticle from nail plate
Nail enamel remover	Acetone or ethyl acetate (solvents), oil, e.g. glycerol (counter drying effect of solvents). Often acetone free now as it is less drying	To gently remove nail enamel
Massage oil/cream	May include: lanolin oils, mineral oils, cetyl alcohol, perfume, preservatives, water	To supplement natural moisture of skin, allow massage movement over skin
Buffing paste	Powdered silica or pumice, wax polish or mineral oil, soft paraffin, paraffin wax	To polish nails, minimise ridges
Nail strengtheners	Formaldehyde	To strengthen nails
Nail enamels, including:base coat, cream, light dark, French manicure and top coat	Plastic film, eg nitrocellulose, plasticiser (for flexibility), solvent for drying), plastic resin (for gloss), pigments (for colour)	To colour, protect and strengthen nails
Pearl and frosted enamels	Guanine or bismuth oxychloride	To colour and decorate nails
Quick driers	Mineral oil and Oleric acid or Silicone	Accelerates the speed at which the polish hardens
Hard skin remover	Sodium chloride, pumice, liquid paraffin and glycerine	To soften and aid in the removal of hard skin

Tool hygiene and sterilisation

It is very important when using tools to maintain high standards of hygiene before, throughout and after treatments.

Note: broken skin around the wall of the cuticle is particularly liable to infection.

See Chapter 1 for information on using autoclaves, UV cabinets and glass bead steriliser and general points on hygiene and sterilisation.

In particular, when using tools for manicures and pedicures:

☐ use a spatula, orange wood stick or cotton bud to remove products from containers

☐ always replace tops on bottles and other products

☐ keep bottle tops clean, so they remain airtight when closed

☐ store prepared tipped orange wood sticks in an airtight container

☐ wipe tools with sanitiser or equivalent after use

☐ place tools in the steriliser after use

☐ after cleaning and sterilisation, store tools hygienically in a chemical sanitiser or UV cabinet (see Chapter 1 for details)

☐ dispose of any waste safely and appropriately.

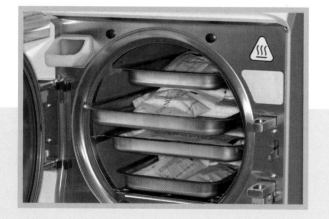

ENDPOINTS
You should now understand:

☐ Contra-actions that may occur during manicure and pedicure

☐ manicure and pedicure tools and their functions

☐ the ingredients and purpose of pedicure and manicure products

☐ pedicure tool hygiene and sterilisation.

Topic 5: Nail shapes, massage and manicure treatments

Nail shaping, nail and cuticle care, hand and arm massage and nail enamelling are the usual elements of a basic manicure treatment.

Client consultation

At the beginning of the manicure, discuss with your client their choice of nail shape and length. Give advice if necessary or if your client asks you, but above all listen to your client's view and abide by their wishes. Similarly, you can advise and suggest colours for enamels, but choice of colour can be very personal and you must follow your client's preferences.

Note: Ask your client about any allergies to products such as hand creams, nail enamels or hardeners and make a note on the client consultation card. Be aware of any adverse reactions (contra-actions), such as redness or itching, to any products used. If these occur, wipe off the product immediately and make a note of it.

Nail shapes

Growth can be affected by:

☐ environment/lifestyle

☐ health

☐ treatment

☐ diet.

☐ climate

☐ damage

Nail shapes can be altered by manicure to suit:

☐ client's preference

☐ fashion

☐ working conditions

☐ shape of the hands

☐ condition of the nail.

The main nail shapes are:

☐ **oval** – best suited to tapered hands; often regarded as the most desirable shape, though this can change with fashion

☐ **square** – the strongest shape, following the shape of the fingertips; usual shape for men, and for people whose jobs require nails to be short, e.g. cooks, health care professionals, therapists

☐ **long square** – especially for French manicure

☐ **pointed** – the weakest shape; generally not advised

☐ **round** – best suited to small, thin hands.

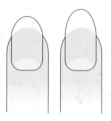

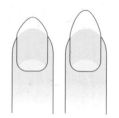

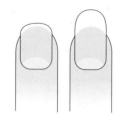

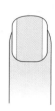

Oval nail

Generally considered to be the most attractive nail shape. Oval nails give the effect of length without producing a fragile point.

Pointed nail

Clients who are impatient for their nails to grow sometimes shape them in to a point so that they look longer. This is the worst thing they could do: a pointed nail will soon snap off.

A square nail

Short, square nails are often preferred by clients because of their jobs, for example people who handle food, and beauty therapists.

Wide nail

Wide nails can be made to appear slimmer by leaving a narrow strip free from enamel at either side of the nail. This creates the illusion of extra length, which draws attention away from the width.

Preparing for manicure

With your prepared manicure tools on a convenient table, manicure trolley or couch, prepare your client.

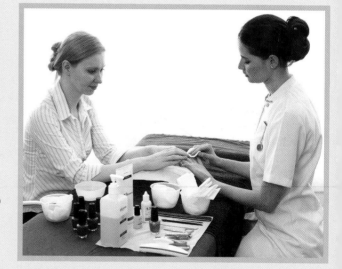

☐ Make sure your client is sitting comfortably in a position they can maintain for the length of the manicure, up to 30 minutes.

☐ Support your client's arm on a cushion on their lap or over the manicure station – it should be relaxed and not stretched.

☐ Place your client's jewellery in a lined bowl on the manicure table or nearby.

☐ If necessary, cover your client's lap with a towel.

☐ Turn back your client's sleeve to the elbow and protect with tissue.

You must also make sure that you are sitting comfortably, not bent over or at an angle and not having to stretch.

Manicure procedure

1. Wipe your client's hands with sanitiser while checking for contraindications.

☐ Remove enamel

☐ Finger rotation should always be used when performing a manicure or pedicure. Always start with the little finger first followed by the thumb then second, third, fourth fingers etc. to ensure that the other nails are not smudged when a procedure is carried out on each nail.

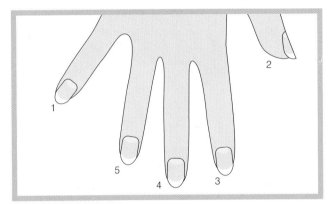

☐ Remove enamel on nails using cotton wool pads soaked in enamel remover held between the fingers to ensure that the manicurist's enamel is not removed in the process. Hold the cotton wool on the nail plate for 3 to 5 seconds to dissolve the enamel then pull the cotton wool forward to the end of the nail plate in order to remove all enamel from the nail plate. Finish using tipped orange wood sticks soaked in remover to clean the cuticle and free edge.

2. File nails. Using an emery board, file the nails on one hand to the shape your client has chosen.

☐ Hold the file at a 45° angle to the nail.

☐ File in one direction only – from the side to the centre, and opposite side to centre. Do not 'saw' the nail.

☐ Follow the shape of the cuticle as a guide.

☐ Do not file the sides lower than the side of the free edge of the nail as this weakens the nail plate and may cause in growing nails.

☐ Finish filing by bevelling the edge of the nail smooth with the fine side of the emery board to prevent nails from splitting, to seal the layers and to remove any rough edges

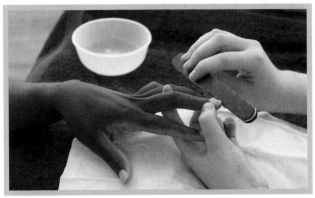

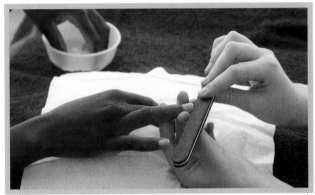

Follow this procedure for each nail as per the finger rotation sequence.

3. Apply cuticle cream.

Using an orange wood stick tipped with cotton wool apply cuticle cream to the cuticles of the filed nails. With firm circular movements, massage the cuticle cream well into the cuticle and surrounding skin of the fingers.

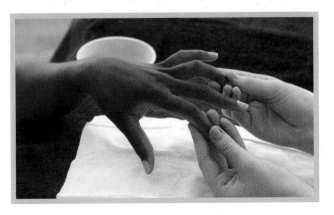

THE ART AND SCIENCE OF BEAUTY THERAPY

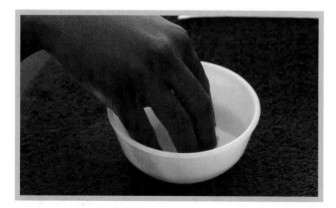

4. Soak the fingertips in the finger bowl.
Soak the massaged fingertips in a bowl of warm soapy water while repeating steps 2 and 3 on the other hand. When that hand is soaking, start cuticle work on the first hand.

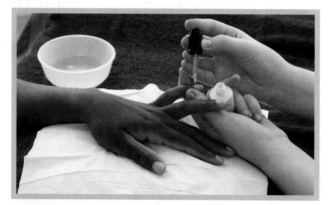

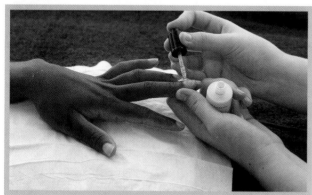

5. Remove the first hand from the water and dry gently with a clean towel or tissues before pushing back the cuticles. Begin the cuticle work

6. Neaten the cuticle. Apply a small amount of cuticle remover then:

☐ using an orange wood stick tipped with cotton wool, gently push the cuticle back using small circular movements

☐ use the hoof stick in small circular movements around the cuticle to push it back off the nail plate

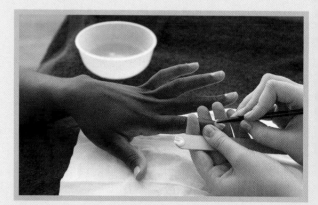

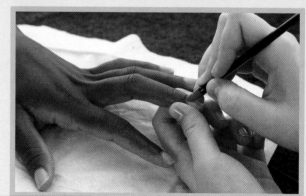

☐ keeping the nail damp, hold the cuticle knife between the thumb, index and middle finger (like a pen) and using a wet cuticle knife at a 45° angle (very low on the nail), gently free any excess cuticle from the nail plate. Work from one side to the centre and then the opposite side to the centre – in small circular movements, never straight across.

☐ wipe away remaining cuticle remover with a wet nail brush or damp cotton wool, pushing the cuticles back as you dry.

Smooth and dry the nail with a towel or tissue. If necessary, and without pulling the skin, cut back dead cuticle/ hangnails cleanly with sanitised cuticle nippers. Never cut the cuticle itself.

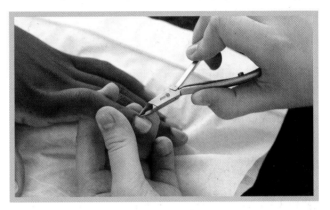

Apply a small amount of hand lotion; wrap the hand in a towel and repeat step 5 and 6 on the other hand.

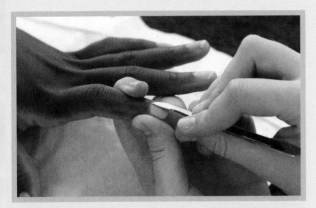

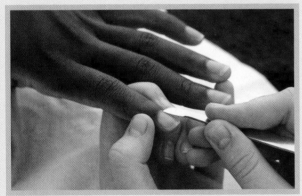

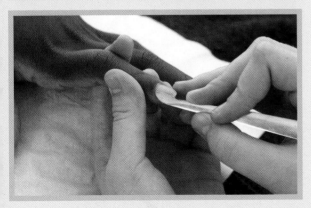

Hand and arm massage

Massage is an integral part of the manicure sequence for several reasons. Hand and arm massage:

- relaxes
- stimulates blood circulation, encouraging nutrients to the area and eliminating waste
- improves skin texture and appearance
- improves joint mobility
- softens and moisturises skin with the massage cream or oil
- helps desquamation.

Contraindications to massage

The contraindications to massage are the same as those for manicures, but be especially aware of:

- skin diseases
- nail diseases
- recent sunburn on arms
- recent scar tissue
- very thin skin
- recent fractures.

Preparing for massage

Having prepared your client for manicure, you just need to make sure that they are still comfortable and the arm is well supported.

Hand cream – see page 98 for details of contents of massage creams and oils.

Massage movements – use the classical massage movements described in Chapter 3:

- Effleurage – stroking
- Petrissage – compression, either of tissue against tissue or tissue against bone
- Passive movements over and around the joints to increase suppleness and mobility. Keep massage strokes smooth and continuous.

Hand and arm massage sequence

Here is a suggested hand and arm massage sequence:

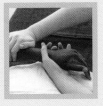 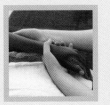 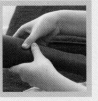 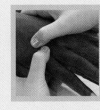 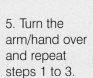

1. Full effleurage covering the whole of the hand and forearm. Repeat six times.

2. Thumb kneading to the anterior forearm in 3 sections covering the whole arm. Repeat six times.

3. Kneading around the carpals. Repeat three times.

4. Kneading in between the metacarpals

5. Turn the arm/hand over and repeat steps 1 to 3.

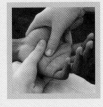 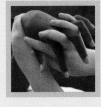 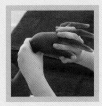

6. Thumb kneading to the palm of the hand

7. Cross frictions to the palm

8. Passive movements with wrist supported. Link the client's fingers and rotate the wrist three times to the left and three times to the right.

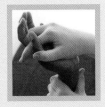 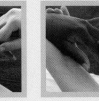 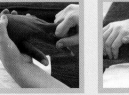 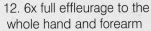

10. Gently flex and extend the wrist

11. Kneading to the phalanges with finger pulls

12. 6x full effleurage to the whole hand and forearm

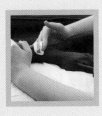

13. Remove massage medium with damp cotton wool

14. Tone the area.

15. Some manicure routines may include use of hot towels for removal of excess product.

16. Squeak the nails – use nail enamel remover to remove any excess oil from the nail plate.

Nail buffing

Nail buffing can be used instead of enamelling, to give a natural, polished look, or as part of the preparation for enamelling. It also concludes a manicure for a male client.

Nail buffing:

☐ improves the appearance of nails

☐ smoothes out superficial ridges

☐ stimulates circulation

☐ removes stains from the nail plate.

Nail buffing technique

1. Remove paste from its container using an orange wood stick, and then replace the lid of the container.

2. Apply a pin-head amount of buffing paste to the centre of each nail.

3. Using the buffer, buff the nail in one direction only – from the matrix to the free edge – the direction in which the nail cells grow, to encourage smoothness of the nail plate.

4. Use regular, rhythmical movements; do not allow the paste to touch the skin tissue.

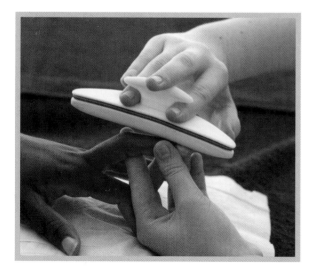

Nail enamelling

If a nail strengthener is used, apply this before applying the base coat.

The base coat:

☐ protects the nail from staining by dark enamels

☐ should be appropriate for the condition of the nail, eg strong, fragile or ridged

☐ gives a smooth surface for enamelling.

1. Apply the base coat to each nail using three even strokes, brushing from the cuticle to the nail tip.

2. Using an orange wood stick or cotton wool bud dipped in nail enamel remover, immediately remove any base coat that gets on to the cuticle or skin.

Nail enamels

There are two types of nail enamel:

Cream – always apply a top coat

Frosted/pearl – top coat not necessary.

Your client will have chosen the type and colour of nail enamel before the start of the manicure.

The manicure treatment should take a maximum of 30 minutes.

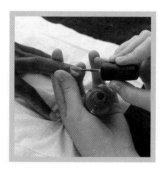
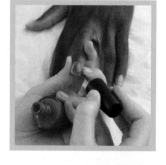
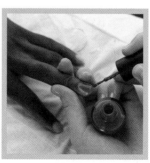
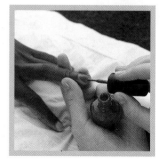

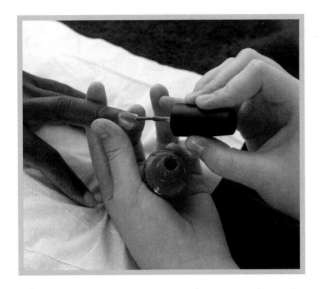

Applying nail enamel

1. Apply the coloured enamel in three strokes per nail.

2. Apply two coats for cream enamels and seal with one coat of top coat. Three coats must be applied for frosted enamels and no top coat should be applied.

3. Apply thinly, to allow each coat to dry more quickly and prevent flaking or chipping.

4. Leave a hairline gap around the nail wall.

5. Ensure no enamel touches the cuticle or skin tissue. If it does, remove it immediately with an orange wood stick or cotton bud dipped in nail enamel remover.

Top coat and drying spray

If a top coat is required, apply in three strokes per nail. The benefits of using a top coat are that it:

☐ seals the enamel

☐ gives extra shine

☐ prevents chipping

☐ increases longevity of the enamel.

A quick drying spray can be used to set the surface of the nail. Always spray away from the client and from furniture. Remember that the underlying layers of enamel will still be soft and that quick dry tends to dry the surface enamel too quickly resulting in premature chipping.

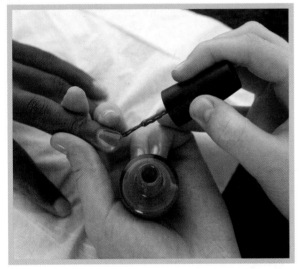

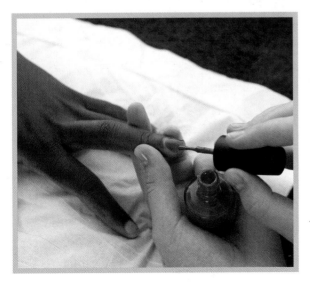

French polish

This has become very popular in recent years. A base coat would be applied as normal followed by a white or cream polish on the free edge of the nail plate to lighten it.

Depending upon the effect the clients requires, either clear, beige or pale pink polish is then applied over the top. Top coat can be applied as normal.

French polish gives a very natural look to the nails and for that reason is particularly popular with brides.

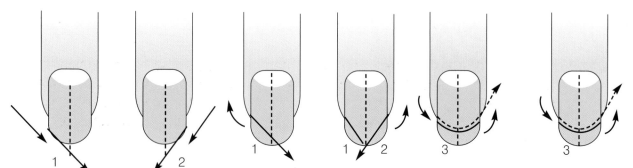

Chevron

The polish is applied down the length of the nail from each side to the opposite corner of the free edge. The point of the chevron sits on the mid line down the length of the nail plate.

Rounded chevron

The chevron is applied first and the 'smile line' is created by sweeping the brush across the nail to round off the point of the chevron and produce a soft curve.

Rounded

the smile line is produced in one sweep of the brush, from side to side, dipping slightly in the middle to produce a soft curve. White polish is applied to the rest of the nail tip, working down the free edge in no more than three brush strokes

Home care advice

Proper home care of nails will prolong the beneficial effects of the professional manicure. You can also give advice to help your client maintain healthy nails and treat underlying problems. See earlier for the underlying reasons for some nail problems. Keep nails protected by:

- using gloves for all household work
- using nail strengtheners, base coat and enamels
- soaking very brittle nails in warm oil
- massaging cuticle cream into nail folds and surrounding skin at night
- applying hand cream after hands have been in water, and last thing at night
- using emery boards, not metal files
- not biting nails or picking at cuticles
- wearing gloves in winter.

ENDPOINTS
You should now understand:

- client consultation
- nail shapes
- preparation for manicure
- manicure procedures
- hand and arm massage procedures
- contraindications to massage
- preparation for massage
- hand and arm massage sequence
- nail buffing
- nail enamelling
- home care advice for manicures.

Topic 6: Specialised treatments and nail enhancements

Specialised treatments and nail enhancement systems can be added to the basic manicure and massage treatment. Specialised treatments are usually arranged if the client needs extra work on, for instance, flaking nails, joint mobility or blood circulation. Nail enhancement systems are different types of nail extensions used to repair or improve the appearance of nails, or for special occasions.

Specialised treatments include:

☐ hot oil

☐ paraffin wax

☐ foot masks

☐ hand masks

☐ exfoliation

☐ thermal mittens/boots.

Nail enhancement systems include:

☐ gels

☐ acrylics

☐ fibre glass

☐ silk wraps

☐ nail art.

Hot oil treatment
Hot oil treatment should use good quality oil, such as almond oil. Before using nut oils, ensure that the client does not have any allergies. The treatment is used to:

☐ moisturise dry skin and cuticles

☐ moisturise flaking nails.

Applying hot oil treatment
1. Follow the manicure procedure and file the nail first.

2. Warm the oil to a comfortable temperature by standing the oil container in a bowl of hot water.

3. Place your client's whole hands, or nails up to the first joint, in a bowl in the warm oil.

4. Allow the hands to soak for 10–15 minutes.

5. Return to the manicure procedure for cuticle work.

Advise your client about using this treatment at home if found to be beneficial.

Paraffin wax
Paraffin wax treatment is used to:

☐ nourish and moisturise the skin – especially beneficial to clients whose skin is cracked and in poor condition; the wax treatment will help absorb nourishing creams into the skin

☐ relieve the pain of stiff joints and improve mobility

☐ improve flaking nail conditions

☐ improve skin colour.

Equipment

☐ A paraffin wax heater, preferably one with a thermostatic control to keep the wax at a temperature of 48–49°C.

☐ Cling film or two large sheets of foil

☐ Large brush

☐ Two towels

☐ Paraffin wax.

Preparations

☐ Cover your client with a gown and the surrounding area with polythene to protect against wax drips.

☐ Place the paraffin wax heater or bath on a secure surface, not a glass trolley or table top.

☐ Follow the instructions for your wax heater, but you will usually need to turn it on about 30 minutes before use.

Applying paraffin wax treatment

1. Apply after filing and before cuticle work. Then swap, and perform cuticle work and hand and arm massage on the waxed hand while the 2nd hand is being given the wax treatment.

2. Always test the temperature of the wax before applying.

3 Hand cream or oil may be applied first then paraffin wax should be brushed onto the hand /foot gradually building it up in layers until it forms a glove

4. Wrap the waxed hand or foot in cling film or foil and then wrap around with a towel to keep the heat in.

5. Leave for about 15 minutes and then unwrap the hand and remove the film/foil and wax together.

The tissues are now in a relaxed state for massage and any excess oil can be incorporated into the treatment.

Wax should be disposed of after use and not re-used. Always keep the lid on the paraffin wax bath when it is not actually being used.

Hand/foot masks

Hand/foot masks are used to draw out impurities and nourish the skin leaving it feeling fresh and soft. Apply after filing the nails.

Start the manicure/pedicure as normal and after the filing:

1. Apply the mask to the hands/feet with a mask brush.

2. Place the hands/feet in towelling mitts/boots or wrap in a towel for about 10 minutes.

3. According to the manufacturer's instructions, rinse off or remove the mask with warm damp towels.

4. Continue with cuticle work

Exfoliators

Exfoliators are gentle, deep-cleansing, abrasive creams that are used to soften rough, dry skin and help remove calluses, ingrained dirt and stains.

1. Gently massage the exfoliating cream into the hands or feet with circular movements.

2. Pay particular attention to rough areas.

3. Rinse off well in warm water or remove all abrasive ingredients with damp hot towels or sponges.

Thermal mittens/ boots

Thermostatically controlled mittens are used to:

☐ improve skin colour by increasing circulation

☐ nourish and hydrate skin and add moisture to the nail plate

☐ soothe aching joints and improve mobility

☐ help remove waste products by improving lymph flow.

Thermal mittens/boots can be used with treatments such as paraffin wax/masks to keep the covered hands warm. They can also be used as a treatment with moisturising products/masks.

Applying thermal mittens/boots
1. Moisturise the hands/foot and nails generously.

2. Wrap hands/feet in cling film.

3. Place hands in thermal mittens at a temperature that is comfortable for your client.

4. Leave for about 10–15 minutes, depending upon the dryness of the skin, before removing and continuing with cuticle work or massage.

Nail enhancement systems

Nail extensions and overlays are now extremely popular, often as specialised treatments on their own. They can be used in the photographic and modelling world, for personal special occasions such as weddings, or for everyday wear. They are also used to improve the appearance of damaged or very short nails, and protect the natural nails as they grow.

Acrylics or gels can be 'sculptured' over a full nail plate or a nail tip attached to the natural nail with glue; fibreglass or silk can be overlaid or 'wrapped' over the natural nail to repair and neaten it. Most important, however, is that they look and feel natural. Your client's occupation or the condition of their nail plate will often suggest the most appropriate system.

☐ Acrylic is harder wearing and so more suitable for clients with manual work, such as gardening.

☐ Fibreglass expands and contracts with water, so is more suitable for clients whose hands are often in water, such as hairdressers.

☐ Silk wraps can give a natural look to nail repairs.

☐ Gel nails protect brittle nails allowing them to grow, but are not as strong as acrylic or fibre-glass systems.

ENDPOINTS
You should now understand:

☐ hot oil treatments

☐ paraffin wax treatments

☐ hand/foot masks

☐ exfoliators

☐ thermal mittens/boots

☐ nail technology systems.

Topic 7: Pedicure treatments

Pedicures are very similar to manicures. They can help to:

- ☐ enhance the appearance of the feet and toe nails

- ☐ nourish the tissues and improve circulation

- ☐ help prevent toenails from splitting, and other minor damage

- ☐ discourage chilblains and help prevent minor foot conditions such as corns, callouses and ingrowing toenails.

Pedicures can therefore give a client more confidence when going barefoot or in sandals, but also alleviate discomfort and help prevent the postural problems that can arise, through making allowances for sore feet.

Contraindications to pedicure

Contraindications to pedicure are the same as for manicures (see page 177) and general contraindications covered in Chapter 1, but in particular be aware of:

- ☐ any nail disease (see Topic 2 for nail diseases)

- ☐ any skin disease, especially tinea pedis 'athlete's foot' or verrucas

- ☐ broken bones

- ☐ swollen toe, ankle or knee joints

- ☐ open cuts or wounds.

Tools and products

These have been discussed earlier, and are similar to those for manicures, but can also include:

- ☐ a pedicure rasp – a tool used to remove hard skin remover, particularly for the balls of the feet and the heels. Hard skin may be removed after the filing has been completed using this implement.

- ☐ a bowl or foot bath large enough for both feet

- ☐ coarse emery boards

- ☐ toenail clippers

- ☐ foot powder

- ☐ foot spray

- ☐ soap and antiseptic

- ☐ disposable paper towels or tissues – the most hygienic way to dry feet and separate toes during enamelling

- ☐ extra towels for wrapping feet.

Note: As with manicure products, always decant products such as creams using a spatula first, and always replace tops on bottles and containers.

Preparing for pedicure

1. Make sure your client is seated in a comfortable chair with back support and you have a low stool or similar which enables you to hold your client's foot in a position comfortable for both of you.

2. Soak the feet in a foot bath/bowl of warm water with antiseptic or foot soak to clean and refresh the feet.

3. Check for contraindications by talking to your client (see Chapter 1 and Topic 2 above) and by a visual check.

4. Give advice to seek medical attention of necessary.

5. Work on one foot while keeping the other foot warm in a towel.

Pedicure technique

1. After removing any enamel with enamel remover, cut the nails straight across with toenail clippers.

2. File the nails straight across and keep them straight to avoid ingrowing toe nails. For the same reason, toenails should not be cut low at the sides or curved.

3. Massage cuticle cream well into the skin around the nail.

4. Soak the foot in warm water, then dry with tissues and wrap in a towel or thermal boot (as above) while working on the other foot.

5. When the second foot has reached stage 5, start cuticle work on the first foot.

6. Remove any hard skin – generally on the balls of the feet and heels – using the hard skin remover tool or the cream massaged into the affected areas. This should only be done on damp skin.

7. Gently push the cuticles back using cuticle remover on cotton wool on an orange wood stick, alternating with the hoof stick/wet nail brush, using small circular movements. Take care to keep the skin intact to prevent infection.

8. Use a wet cuticle knife in small circular movements, flat against the nail, to loosen dead tissue.

9. Dry the nails with tissue/towel, and if necessary carefully cut any dead cuticle remaining on the nail with dry cuticle clippers.

10. Wrap the foot in a towel and apply a nourishing cream, then wrap the foot in a towel.

11. Repeat steps 7–10 with the other foot.

Pedicure massage technique

Massage technique for the foot and lower leg is very similar to that for the hand and arm described earlier. As well as friction movements, you can use the classical massage movements of:

☐ **effleurage** – stroking

☐ **petrissage** – compression

☐ **tapotement** – percussion

☐ **passive** – movements to increase mobility in the joints.

Preparing for the massage

Before beginning a massage sequence, your client should be prepared:

☐ Your client should be sitting in a well-supported chair.

☐ Make sure your client's leg is well supported and not uncomfortably extended.

☐ Apply oil, lotion or massage cream as far as the knee.

The foot and leg massage sequence

Here is one example of how to combine the movements in a pedicure massage:

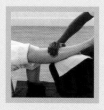 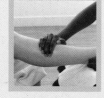 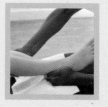 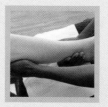 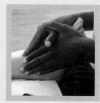

1.6x Effleurage to whole leg and foot

2.6x kneading to the medial aspect of the gastrocnemius

3.6x stroking around the ankle

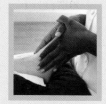 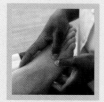 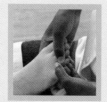 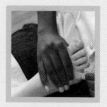 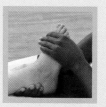

4.6x stroking over the whole foot

5. Thumb kneading between the phalanges

6. Thumb kneading to the metatarsals

7. Rotate the toes each way individually

8. Passive movements – rotate the ankle each way – point and flex twice

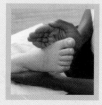 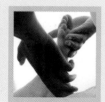 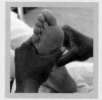 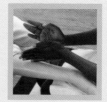 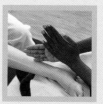 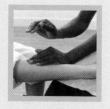

9. Stroking to the instep (medial side)

10. Palmar stroking to the sole of the foot

11. Cross friction to the sole of the foot

12. Hacking on the gastrocnemius

13. Cupping on the gastrocnemius

  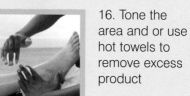

14.6x effleurage to the whole leg and foot

15. Remove massage medium with damp cotton wool

16. Tone the area and or use hot towels to remove excess product

17. Squeak the nails – wipe over with nail enamel remover to remove any surplus massage oil.

Enamelling the toenails

Your client may want their toes enamelled as a beauty treatment on its own or as part of the pedicure. Discuss this before the pedicure and allow the client to choose the enamel before you start.

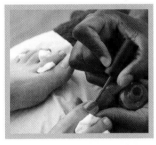

1. Place tissues between the toes to keep them apart and avoid smudging the enamel.

2. The foot must be flat so that the enamel does not run back onto the cuticles.

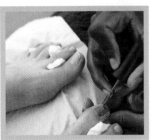

3. Clean the nails with enamel remover, apply a base coat, two coats of enamel and one coat of top coat. For more details, see the topic on manicures.

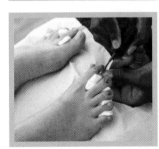

4. When the enamel is dry, remove the tissues from between the toes. The client may then put their footwear back on, however they should be advised to bring open toed shoes.

Always clean, sterilise or safely dispose of tools used in pedicure treatments. The pedicure procedure should be kept within the 40 minutes time limit acceptable to the industry.

Home care advice

Give advice to your clients about keeping their feet in good condition. This may include:

☐ keeping feet mobile: picking up a pencil with the toes is a good foot exercise; many foot exercises can be done while sitting down, such as stretching and relaxing legs and feet

☐ walking barefoot will tone the muscles and ligaments

☐ lose weight, if necessary, as excess weight can put undue pressure on the feet

☐ only wear correctly fitting shoes, high heel shoes are not good for posture

☐ use foot products, such as foot sprays and powders, to keep feet refreshed and healthy and prevent infection

☐ soak feet in foot baths with Epsom salts or sea salt to draw moisture out of swollen or aching feet

☐ massage the feet often, as this is good for the whole body as well as the feet.

Client record card

Always keep your client record card up to date with each visit, noting the condition of the feet, contraindications, treatments given, products used and any contra-actions, and any advice or aftercare guidance that you have given your client.

ENDPOINTS
You should now understand:

☐ the contraindications to pedicures

☐ pedicure tools and products

☐ how to prepare for a pedicure

☐ pedicure techniques

☐ pedicure massage techniques

☐ how to enamel the toenails

☐ home care advice for pedicures

☐ the need to maintain the client record card for pedicures.

Chapter 6: Depilation

introduction

Depilation, or temporary hair removal, like many other beauty treatments, has been affected by technological advances.

Although waxing techniques have been used for many years, recent adaptations to these methods mean that they are now quicker, safer, and more hygienic than they once were. Hair removal, for both men and women, and from all parts of the body, is also more popular than in the past. Most salons provide this treatment, while some specialise exclusively in depilation.

Topic 1: Anatomy and physiology of the hair

In Chapter 2 we looked in some detail at the structure and functions of the skin. In this topic we will look more closely at hair – how it is structured and how it grows.

Structure and function of hair

Hair grows in follicles which are in the dermis, the layer of skin beneath the epidermis. See Chapter 2 for more details of the skin and its structure. The dermis is connected to the blood and lymph supply as well as the nerves. It is made up of connective tissue, containing sweat glands, sebaceous glands and hair follicles.

Hair follicles

The hair follicles travel through the epidermis and the dermis. The erector pili muscles are attached to each hair and help with temperature control of the body by pulling the hair upright and trapping a layer of air – goose pimples to keep the body warm (vasoconstriction).

Sebaceous glands

Associated with each hair follicle is a sebaceous gland. These produce sebum, a fatty acid which keeps the skin moist and lubricates the hair shaft. When sweat and sebum combine on the surface of the skin they form the acid mantle, a protective shield which helps to control bacteria levels, prevents infections and disease, and acts as a natural moisturiser. The pH balance of the skin is 4.5 –5.6 and this acid environment helps to prevent bacterial growth.

CROSS-SECTION OF THE HAIR IN THE FOLICLE

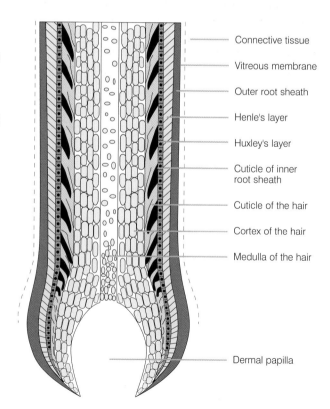

- Connective tissue
- Vitreous membrane
- Outer root sheath
- Henle's layer
- Huxley's layer
- Cuticle of inner root sheath
- Cuticle of the hair
- Cortex of the hair
- Medulla of the hair
- Dermal papilla

Types of hair

The hair growing on a human body can be one of three different types, depending on how old the person is and where the hair is growing.

Lanugo hair

About six months before a child is born, it begins to develop a coat of fine, soft, downy hair all over its body. These hairs begin growing at the same time, and grow at the same rate. The lanugo hair is normally shed one month before the child is born, but premature babies may be born still covered in lanugo hair.

Vellus hairs

The follicles that produce vellus hairs have no sebaceous glands, and are distributed over most of the body, with the exception of the soles of the feet, palms of the hands, the lips and nipples. Pale in colour, vellus hairs themselves only grow to one to two centimetres in length.

Terminal hairs

What we normally think of as hair is called terminal hair, and is produced by hair follicles with sebaceous glands. It grows on the head, areas of the face, underarms and the pubic area. Congenital tendencies to baldness may result in terminal hairs becoming shorter and thinner, so that they resemble vellus hairs.

Hair growth cycle

The hair that we so often describe as 'growing' is actually mostly dead. The hair grows at its base, the hair bulb, in the follicle, and the hair we see above about a centimetre from the skin is in fact a dead shaft of keratin. The hair will grow from its base in the follicle for many years, and then falls out. The follicle rests for a while, and then resumes production of a new hair. This hair growth cycle has three stages, called the Anagen, Catogen and Telogen.

Anagen

The anagen, or growing, phase can last from two to seven years, during which time the hair grows vigorously, at a rate of about a centimetre per month, although the hair can grow more quickly in the summer. Untrimmed, each of our hairs would grow to about a metre long before falling out! During the anagen phase, the hair bulb generates the pigment melanin, which gives our hair its colour. The length of the anagen stage of the cycle is an inherited characteristic.

Catagen

The anagen phase is followed by a phase of two to four weeks when the follicle rests. This phase is called the catagen, or intermediate, phase. The bulb produces neither hair cells nor pigment, and shrinks slightly, becoming less deep.

Telogen

In the telogen phase a new hair begins to grow in the hair follicle. As it does so, the old hair will be shed as we brush or wash our hair. By the end of the telogen phase, which lasts about three months, the old hair has been shed, and a new one is growing from the follicle and out of the skin, ready to begin its own anagen phase.

Factors that affect the hair growth cycle

A range of factors can affect hair growth. These factors may be hormonal, dietary, environmental or, as we saw when discussing the hair growth cycle, they may be hereditary.

Hormonal factors

As we will see in the next topic on the endocrine system, there are a variety of hormonal factors that affect the hair growth cycle. As the state of the endocrine system changes as an individual grows, and varies according to stress, menstrual cycles, etc., the hair growth cycle is also affected.

Changes in androgen (male hormone) levels particularly affect the hair, and affect the rate of hair growth and the thickness of the hairs.

Female hormone levels (oestrogens) slow hair growth and extend the growing phase of the hair growth cycle.

As a result, hair growth can be affected in several ways by the balance of androgens and oestrogen in the blood. At the time of puberty the rise in androgen levels is responsible for the hair on the body changing into recognisable terminal hair, and the development of underarm and pubic hair. Later in life, changes in hormone levels will increase face, chest, nose and ear hair growth. In women, hair growth can be affected by hormonal changes during pregnancy, when they have high levels of oestrogen. and during the menopause when the oestrogen levels reduce.

Other hormones can also affect the hair, e.g. thyroid hormone accelerating hair growth.

Diet and environmental factors

Hair growth can be affected by both general diet, and specific dietary deficiencies. A very poor diet can lead to hair loss, through its effect on the endocrine system, and the changes of hormone levels that it induces. This can be seen in people who go on crash diets, or those who suffer from anorexia. Problems may also be caused by factors as varied as anaemia, alcohol consumption, or a lack of Vitamin B or zinc in a diet.

ENDPOINTS
By the end of this topic, you should understand:

☐   the structure and function of hair

☐   the types of hair

☐   the hair growth cycle

☐   the factors that affect the hair growth cycle.

Topic 2:
The Endocrine system

The endocrine system is one of the body's communication systems. The endocrine system is composed of ductless glands that produce hormones, the body's chemical messengers, which it uses to tell the body what to do. Hormones control and affect many body functions and organs, as well as behaviour. Each gland produces specific hormones. The function of the endocrine system is closely linked to that of the nervous system.

The structure and function of the endocrine system

What is a hormone?

A hormone is a chemical messenger, which is secreted directly into the blood by a particular gland. Some hormones, such as insulin, are made of protein, but others are steroids (adreno-corticoid hormones), glycoproteins (FSH, LH, TSH), and derivatives of single amino acids, (T4, T3). Hormones are produced in the gland and are then transported to the area/organ they control or affect.

What is an endocrine gland?

An endocrine gland is a ductless gland which produces hormones. Ductless means that there is no separate canal or tube to transport the hormones to the blood. Hormones travel straight into the bloodstream from the gland.

What do hormones and the endocrine system do?

They affect the behaviour and function of different areas of the body and of the body overall, e.g. hormones are responsible for correct growth, changes during puberty, the menstrual cycle, pregnancy, the menopause, responses to stress and danger and the proper functioning of the kidneys and digestive system.

The main glands of the body

The diagram below shows the main endocrine glands of the body and lists the hormones secreted. The following section explains the function and malfunction of each hormone. If too much of a hormone is produced it is known as hypersecretion, whereas the production of too little is known as hyposecretion.

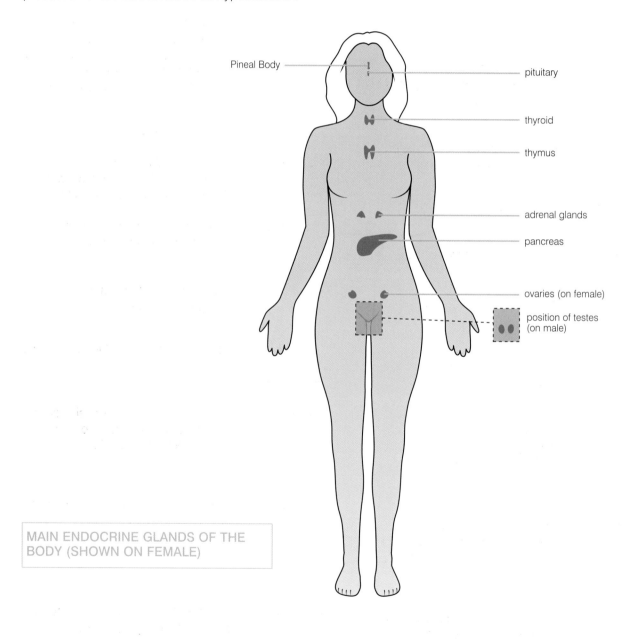

Pineal Body

pituitary

thyroid

thymus

adrenal glands

pancreas

ovaries (on female)

position of testes (on male)

MAIN ENDOCRINE GLANDS OF THE BODY (SHOWN ON FEMALE)

The endocrine glands and their hormones

This section explains the functions and malfunctions of the glands and hormones.

PITUITARY

Location: Situated at the base of the brain, closely connected to the hypothalamus; has two hormone-secreting lobes, the anterior and posterior.

Anterior lobe hormones

Human growth hormone (HGH)

Function: regulates height and growth; main controller along with the genes of the final height of a person

Melanocyte-stimulating hormone (MSH)

Function: stimulates production of melanin in the basal layer of the skin.

Thyrotrophin (TSH)

Function: controls the thyroid gland

Adrenocorticotrophin (ACTH)

Function: controls the adrenal cortex

Prolactin or lactogenic hormone (LTH)

Function: production of milk during lactation.

Gonadotrophins (gonad/sex organ hormones)

Function: controls sexual development and organs (ovaries and testes)

Follicle-stimulating hormone (FSH)

Function: stimulates ovaries to produce oestrogen and to ovulate in women and stimulates sperm production in men.

Luteinising hormone (LH)

Function: stimulates ovaries to produce the corpus luteum from the ruptured follicle and produce progesterone.

Interstitial cell-stimulating hormone (ICSH)/luteinising hormone in men

Function: stimulates sperm production and secretion of testosterone.

Posterior lobe hormones

Antidiuretic hormone (ADH or vasopressin)

Function: regulates water absorption in the kidneys

Oxytocin

Function: contracts mammary glands when suckling begins, to release the milk secreted into the ducts; contraction of muscles of the uterus to begin childbirth and during the process.

Thyroid glands

Location: either side of the neck

Hormones: thyroxin, triiodothyronine and calcitonin produced in response to TSH (from pituitary, anterior lobe).

Functions: stimulate tissue metabolism; maintain BMR (basic metabolic rate).

Calcitonin

Function: maintenance of calcium and phosphorus balance.

Parathyroids

Location: four, two either side behind the thyroid.

Hormones: parathormone

Functions: maintenance of calcium level in plasma; stimulates calcium reabsorption in kidneys; activates Vitamin D.

ADRENAL GLANDS

Location: one on top of each kidney NB: split into two parts, adrenal cortex and adrenal medulla

Adrenal cortex

Mineralocorticoids – aldosterone (steroids)

Function: regulates the salts in the body, especially sodium chloride and potassium.

Glucocorticoids (steroids) (cortisol and cortisone)

Functions: produced in response to ACTH (from pituitary, anterior lobe); metabolises carbohydrates, fats and proteins.

Sex hormones (steroids);

female: oestrogen and progesterone (some normal in male)

male: testosterone (small amounts secreted in the ovaries in females)

Functions: sexual development and maturity; ovulation; hair growth in pubic and axillary (armpit) areas.

Adrenal medulla

The adrenal medulla functions to support the sympathetic nervous system.

Hormones:

Adrenaline and noradrenaline

Function: often known as the stress hormones, they prepare the body for 'fight or flight' by speeding up heart rate, slowing digestive and urinary systems, increasing blood pressure and blood sugar level. Adrenaline is a powerful vasoconstrictor i.e. it constricts blood vessels in order to increase blood pressure.

PANCREAS

(specifically in the islets of Langerhans, specialised cells that form the endocrine part of the pancreas)

Location: behind and slightly below stomach, between duodenum and spleen, connected to the duodenum by the pancreatic duct

Hormone: insulin and glucogen

Function: helps glucose enter cells thus - regulating blood sugar levels.

OVARIES

Location: either side of the uterus

Hormones: female sex hormones – oestrogen and progesterone (the testes produce a small amount in males)

Functions: responsible for fem-ale sexual characteristics e.g. breast growth, widening of hips, pubic and axillary hair growth.

TESTES

Location: within the scrotum, behind the penis

Hormone: male sex hormone – testosterone (the ovaries produce a small amount in females)

Functions: responsible for male sexual characteristics thus sperm production, changes at puberty — voice breaking, pubic, facial and axillary hair growth, increased muscle mass.

PINEAL GLAND/BODY

Location: centre of the brain

Hormone: melatonin (derived from serotonin)

Function: controls body rhythms – responds to sunlight

THYMUS

Location: in the thorax

Hormone: TF and THF, which appear to promote development of T lymphocytes in the thymus gland

Functions: part of the immune system

The role of sex hormones

This section explains the role of sex hormones in the development and function of the body.

Puberty

Puberty is the age at which the internal reproductive organs of boys and girls reach maturity and become functional. Although the effect on these organs cannot be seen, the effect on the rest of the body can, in the form of secondary sexual characteristics. The average age for girls to reach puberty is 10–14, though in some cases it begins as early as 8–9. For boys the average age is 13–16.

The effects of hormones in puberty

In girls, the ovaries are stimulated by two hormones: follicle-stimulating hormone (FSH) and luteinising hormone (LH). These are known as gonadotrophins and they are secreted by the anterior lobe of the pituitary. They have the following effects:

- uterus, fallopian tubes and ovaries reach maturity and become functional ovulation and the menstrual cycle begin
- growth of pubic and axillary hair
- glandular tissue in the breasts enlarges and develops
- increase in height and pelvic width
- increase in amount of subcutaneous fat.

In boys, the same gonadotrophins are produced (follicle-stimulating hormone (FSH) and luteinising hormone (LH), though luteinising hormone is called interstitial cell stimulating hormone (ICSH) in men and it stimulates the testes to produce testosterone. Most of the changes produced are caused by testosterone and the effects are:

- growth of bone and muscle
- noticeable height increase
- the larynx enlarges and the voice breaks
- growth of pubic, facial, axillary, abdominal and chest hair
- development of sexual organs
- the seminiferous tubules in the testes, begin to produce testosterone and sperm.

When does the menstrual cycle stop happening?

Once the menarche (start of menstruation) has passed menstruation only stops in three instances: the onset of amenorrhea (see Diseases and Disorders for more information), pregnancy or the menopause.

Menopause (climacteric)

A woman can, technically speaking, bear children as long as she is menstruating. This reproductive period lasts about 35 years, until the ova (egg) supply is exhausted. Women are born with a certain number of eggs. When these run out, the menopause begins. The average age for menopause to begin is 45-55 and it takes an average of five years to complete (though it can last ten). During this period the hormonal changes that began with puberty will be reversed. For example the ovaries will gradually stop responding to FSH and LH, the hormones that provoked changes in puberty, and thus produce less oestrogen and progesterone. The reduction in these hormones causes irregular menstrual cycles (before menstruation stops completely), shrunken breasts, flushes, sweats, palpitations, atrophied sex organs and, possibly, unpredictable behaviour. Many of the symptoms of the menopause can be alleviated by the use of Hormone Replacement Therapy (HRT). Due to the imbalance of the sex hormones at this time, facial hair growth is stimulated.

Diseases and disorders of the endocrine system

Addison's syndrome

Cause: hyposecretion of adrenocortical hormones (sex, growth and salt regulation hormones).

Effects: muscular atrophy and weakness; hypotension; gastric problems like vomiting, changes in skin pigmentation, irregular menstrual cycle and dehydration.

Amenorrhoea

Cause: can be caused by hypersecretion of testosterone (in females), stress; radical weight loss, anaemia.

Effect: absence of menstruation.

Cushing's syndrome

Cause: hypersecretion of adrenocortical hormones (sex, growth and salt regulation hormones) i.e. the opposite of Addison's syndrome.

Effects: muscular atrophy and weakness, hypertension, moon shaped face, redistribution of body fat, sometimes mental illness, osteoporosis.

Pre-menstrual syndrome

Cause: onset of menstruation; usually occurs about one week before.

Effects: depression, irritability, bloating, swollen and tender breast tissue, restlessness.

Polycystic ovarian syndrome (also known as Stein-Leventhal syndrome)

Cause: not known.

Effects: irregular menstrual cycle, due to excessive stimulation of the ovaries by secretion of luteinising hormone, multiple growth of follicular ovarian cysts and sometimes infertility, enlarged ovaries and often high levels of oestrogen; 50% of patients are obese and become hirsute; age range of sufferers is usually 16-30.

Stress

Stress is a threat to the body and the body responds to it like any other danger – the adrenal medulla releases adrenaline and noradrenaline to help us with the fight or flight response. The physical manifestations of the arrival of adrenaline in the body are faster heart rate and breathing, sweating (hence sweaty palms when we are frightened or nervous), a glucose rush from the liver and heightened senses (like hearing and sight). Prolonged stress may cause amenorrhoea and hirsutism in women and low production of sperm in men.

Interrelationships with other body systems

The endocrine system links other body systems such as the:

☐ **Nervous system:** works very closely with the nervous system to provide homeostasis – balance in the body. The pituitary gland (endocrine) has an infinite link to the hypothalamus (nervous system/brain) both of which exert great control over the body.

☐ **Circulatory system:** hormones are secreted and carried in the bloodstream to the various target organs.

☐ **Reproductive system:** governs the reproductive system particularly in females as it controls the menstrual cycle and the release of hormones during pregnancy and childbirth.

ENDPOINTS

At the end of this topic you should now know about:

☐ the position of the endocrine glands

☐ the names and effects of hormones secreted by each gland

☐ the role of sex hormones in menstruation, pregnancy and menopause

☐ diseases and disorders of the endocrine system.

Topic 3: Preparations for depilation

Clients may want some form of depilation (temporary hair removal) for many different reasons. Whatever the reason, they will want to know that the service is confidential, professional and entirely safe. How you communicate with your client, the preparations you make and the appearance of your salon should reassure them on all these counts.

Communicating with your client

It is important to discuss this very personal treatment with great sensitivity. Look back at Chapter 1 for more information on how to communicate effectively with your client. You will need to consult about the extent of treatment the client wants: for instance, removal of hair from:

☐ the face, eg upper lip, eyebrows, chin

☐ lower legs or full legs

☐ a bikini wax or a Brazilian/Hollywood

☐ the underarms

☐ the forearms

☐ the chest

☐ the abdomen

☐ the back.

You will then need to offer your client the method of treatment suitable for that part of the body, explaining:

☐ what procedures would be necessary for each

☐ the advantages and disadvantages of each method

☐ the time that each method would take

☐ the cost.

It is also important to take a medical history to decide whether there are any contraindications to the treatment, and to give advice where necessary. We shall cover all these topics in this chapter.

When you have consulted with your client and carried out a visual check to see the extent and nature of the hair growth to be removed, you and your client will be able to decide on the most appropriate treatment. You must also keep careful notes, especially of any contraindications, on the client's record card, which you will update after the procedure.

If during the consultation you establish that the client tends to be allergic or sensitive to products, it is advisable to conduct a patch test prior to the waxing treatment.

Advantages and disadvantages of depilation treatments

The depilation treatments are:

☐ hot wax

☐ cool wax

☐ tweezing, sugaring, depilation machines, shaving, creams and threading.

Waxing treatments (the treatments used in professional salons) work by covering the hairs to be removed with wax, which sticks to the hairs. When it is removed, it pulls the hairs out leaving the skin smooth. Tweezing, shaving and depilatory creams are rarely used in salons, but you should know how to advise a client for home use.

When your client has told you which areas of the body they would like treated, it is important to make a visual check before deciding which treatment is most appropriate (see Topic 1 above). This is necessary because, as well as some methods being more

Contraindications requiring medical permission

In circumstances where medical permission cannot be obtained clients must give their informed consent in writing prior to the treatment:

- ☐ Cardio vascular conditions (thrombosis, phlebitis, hypertension, hypotension, heart conditions)
- ☐ Haemophilia
- ☐ Any condition already being treated by a GP or another practitioner
- ☐ Medical oedema
- ☐ Osteoporosis
- ☐ Nervous/Psychotic conditions
- ☐ Recent operations
- ☐ Diabetes
- ☐ Trapped/Pinched nerve
- ☐ Inflamed nerve
- ☐ Severe varicose veins

Contraindications that restrict treatment

- ☐ Fever
- ☐ Infectious or contagious diseases
- ☐ Under the influence of recreational drugs or alcohol
- ☐ Any known allergies
- ☐ Infectious skin diseases and disorders
- ☐ Undiagnosed lumps and bumps
- ☐ Localised swelling
- ☐ Inflammation
- ☐ Cuts, bruises, abrasions
- ☐ Scar tissues (2 years for major operation and 6 months for a small scar)
- ☐ Sunburn
- ☐ Self tan
- ☐ Heat rash
- ☐ Hairy moles
- ☐ Hormonal implants
- ☐ Recent fractures (minimum 3 months)
- ☐ Neuralgia
- ☐ Hypersensitive skin
- ☐ Loss of skin sensation
- ☐ Vascular skin
- ☐ Varicose veins
- ☐ 48 hours after sun tanning
- ☐ Bells Palsy
- ☐ Abnormal hair growth.

appropriate for some areas of the body than others, the length and type of hair growth (for instance, dark, thick coarse hair) will also help determine the most appropriate method.

The advantages of hot wax treatment
- ☐ it is often considered best at treating deep-rooted, coarse, dark hairs and very short hairs (minimum 1cm) as it has the greatest adhering power
- ☐ it is very efficient in treating small areas, such as lip and chin, underarm, bikini
- ☐ the results may last up to six weeks depending upon individual hair growth with regular treatment
- ☐ regrowth is tapered and smooth, not blunt like shaved hairs.

The disadvantages of hot wax treatment:
- ☐ it is put on in thick layers and must be disposed of after each client's use, for hygiene and safety

- ☐ it takes longer to heat up as it must be used at a higher temperature than cool wax
- ☐ it takes longer to cover large areas, such as the back or legs
- ☐ it can be messy if not carefully applied
- ☐ training and proficiency are very important when dealing with hot wax
- ☐ skin reaction may occur due to the higher working temperature.
- ☐ it is not possible to go over the same area more than once.

The advantages of cool wax treatment:
- ☐ the wax reaches the correct temperature more quickly than hot wax
- ☐ the lower temperature is more suitable to sensitive skins and larger areas such as the legs/arms
- ☐ the technique can cover large areas quickly

- ☐ it uses less wax, so is more economical
- ☐ it is clean and easy to use
- ☐ regrowth is tapered and smooth
- ☐ regrowth takes up to 6 weeks depending upon individual hair growth

The disadvantages of cool wax treatment

- ☐ it is less effective in removing dark coarse hairs as efficiently as the hot wax method as they may break
- ☐ removal can be sticky if not performed proficiently
- ☐ it is sometimes uncomfortable
- ☐ hairs need to be longer for effective removal
- ☐ it may cause ingrowing hairs if not performed correctly.

Tweezing, sugaring, depilation machines, shaving creams and threading

- ☐ **Tweezing** – tweezers are used to extract individual hairs from the follicle by tweezing in the direction of growth. This method is used in salons only for shaping eyebrows and for taking out any stray hairs left after waxing. Hairs may grow back darker and coarser.

- ☐ **Sugaring** – Sugar depilation treatments have been used in the Middle East for many years originally developed as a method used at home by Middle Eastern women. Modern professional products, the use of natural products and its gentle but efficient application make sugaring an increasingly popular method of depilation particularly suitable for sensitive skins. Being water soluble, it is also easy to remove from most surfaces by wiping over with a damp cloth. There are two types of sugaring treatment, strip sugar and paste sugar.

Strip sugar is applied in exactly the same way as cool wax, but the product itself needs slightly different preparation. Strip sugar comes in a container, which may be heated in its own heater or a microwave. Always follow the manufacturer's instructions for heating. The texture of the sugar when applied should be runny but not watery. Always test the temperature of the sugar on your wrist and on the client's wrist or ankle before applying. Removal is carried out with paper or muslin strips.

Paste sugar is applied in more traditional ways, using the hands, and needs specialist training. The paste can be heated in tubs in either its own heater or a microwave. It comes as either soft or hard paste, but it must be soft and pliable when used, not runny, sticky or too hard. Paste sugar adapts to outside temperatures quickly, so should be kept in its container with the lid closed in a cool, dry place. Have a bowl of water or damp towel handy in case your hands become sticky with the paste.

- ☐ **Shaving** – an electrical or wet razor is used with soap, cream, oil or gel to cut hairs off at or just below skin level. It is a very short-term depilatory method, with hairs regrowing with coarse, blunt tips, apparent as stubble in about 24 hours. Shaving is not encouraged nor used in salons.

- ☐ **Depilatory creams** – applied with a spatula, left, then removed with a spatula and the cream and hair washed away. These creams contain chemicals which dissolve the hair from slightly below the skin's surface. However, if used regularly, it could cause the skin to become over sensitive, as the chemical is a keratolytic, which attacks the keratin in skin as well as hair. It is not generally used in salons, and specialised depilatory creams must be used on the face.

- ☐ **Threading** – an Asian method of hair removal developed for use at home. Hair is removed by wrapping a thread around the hairs and swiftly pulling them out.

- ☐ **Depilation machines** – a mechanical method of tweezing used for larger areas, mainly the lower legs.

Ingredients in depilation products

Hot wax ingredients

- ☐ beeswax – true wax from the honeycomb, may be yellow, brown or green

- ☐ resins – give the wax flexibility

- ☐ soothing agent or antibacterials – eg azulene, tea tree oil, chamomile or aloe vera.

Cool wax ingredients

- ☐ wax – either organic substances, eg honey or glucose syrup; paraffin wax or rubber latex solution

- ☐ synthetic resins can be added to improve texture and quality

- ☐ healing, antiseptic agents such as tea tree oil or witch hazel can be added.

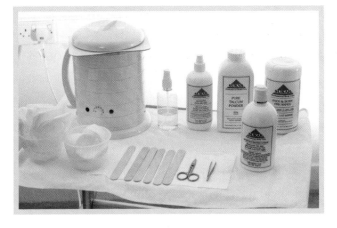

Waxing equipment

The equipment for most treatments, apart from the hot wax machine and the cool wax machine, is very similar and usually includes:

- ☐ sanitiser to cleanse skin

- ☐ pre-wax lotion/gel

- ☐ cotton wool

- ☐ disposable spatulas

- ☐ surgical gloves and apron

- ☐ surgical spirit, or other antiseptic

- ☐ soothing, after-treatment lotion/gel/oil

- ☐ tweezers

- ☐ scissors to trim longer hairs first

- ☐ waste bin

- ☐ separate bin for contaminated waste

- ☐ protect the couch and floor

- ☐ modesty towel for client.

In addition:

- ☐ hot wax treatment uses talcum powder to dry and lift hairs

- ☐ cool wax strips use muslin or paper strips to remove the wax substance and hairs.

Alternatively, salons may use cool wax roll-on applicator systems with detachable or disposable roller heads, which are hygienic and convenient alternatives to using spatulas.

Cool wax, pre-waxed strips, which are available for home use, are not suitable for professional treatments as they are not efficient enough.

Check list
Use this checklist to make sure that you have the correct supplies available before each client session.

Equipment	Hot wax Treatment	Cool wax Treatment
Hot wax machine	●	
Cool wax machine		●
Sanitiser – to cleanse skin	●	●
Talcum powder to dry and lift hairs	●	
Pre-wax lotion or gel	●	●
Cotton wool	●	●
Disposable spatulas	●	●
Muslin or paper strips to remove wax		●
Soothing after-treatment lotion/gel/oil	●	●
Gloves and apron	●	●
Tweezers	●	●
Scissors to trim longer hairs first	●	●
Waste bin	●	●
Separate bin for contaminated waste	●	●
Plastic covers for couch and floor	●	●
Modesty towel for client	●	●

Health and safety – using equipment

The combination of electrical equipment and hot/cool wax should be treated as a potential health and safety hazard and all precautions taken to make sure they are used safely for your client, yourself and your salon. You must ensure that:

☐ all wax machines comply with Safety Standards

☐ heating elements are enclosed, properly wired and have no bare wires

☐ there are no trailing wires in the salon

☐ all wax heating appliances are on trolleys away from anything inflammable

☐ there is no water in the area

☐ wax machines are not moved when hot

☐ you regularly check the temperature of the wax, even on thermostatically controlled machines

☐ machines are cleaned immediately after use with specialist cleaning equipment solution or sanitiser

☐ lids are left on while the machines are not in use.

Safety

Never re-use wax that has been used in a depilation treatment. It should always be disposed of safely and hygienically after use.

ENDPOINTS

By the end of this topic, you should understand:

☐ the contraindications to depilation

☐ the advantages and disadvantages of the depilation treatments

☐ tweezing, sugaring, depilation machines, shaving creams and threading

☐ the ingredients in depilation products

☐ waxing equipment

☐ health and safety aspects of using depilation equipment.

Topic 4: Hot and cool wax treatments

Preparing for all depilation treatments

Having decided which treatment you are going to use, the initial preparations are very similar for all treatments.

Safety: Wax may drip!

1. Prepare your area by protecting the floor and couch.

2. Even more important, make sure that you will not be dripping wax onto any other part of your client than that to be waxed, and that:

    – both your client and your client's clothes are fully protected with paper sheeting or towels

    – the client lies with the part of the body to be waxed closest to the wax pot.

3. Therapists **must** wear gloves

4. Make sure that everything you will need for the treatment is easily to hand and positioned safely.

5. Make sure that the wax is ready at the correct temperature.

6. Check the direction of hair growth. This is important, and is dependant on the type of wax being applied, as hairs should be removed against direction of growth. In some areas, the direction of growth may change several times, for instance on the underarm.

7. Wipe over the area to be treated with sanitiser or other pre-wax lotions.

8. Test the heated wax first on your wrist to check the temperature, and then on your client's wrist or ankle, to make sure it is not too hot.

9. Reassure your client by explaining what you will be doing, any possible reactions and how you will treat these.

Hot wax treatment

1. Apply powder against the hair growth to lift the hairs away from the skin to help them adhere to the wax.

2. Heat the wax to approximately 68°C – always follow the manufacturer's instructions.

3. After testing the temperature first on the therapist and then on the client apply the wax with a disposable spatula held at right angles to the area to be waxed.

4. Apply the wax, against the hair growth, then in the direction of the hair growth, then against it in a figure of eight, building up the edges to ensure they do not break on removal.

5. Build up several layers in strips, leaving similar sized strips in between, so that you can cover the whole area in two sets of strips "chequer board" or, for smaller areas, treat a patch at a time.

3	6
5	2
1	4

6. As the wax is beginning to set, flick up the end that you will use to remove the wax, remembering that you will 'rip' the wax against the direction of hair growth.

7. When the wax has set but is still warm, grip the lifted end and, whilst holding your client's skin taut with your free hand, 'rip' the strip off in one firm, quick action.

8. Immediately place your gloved hand firmly on the waxed area (do not rub). This lessens the stinging sensation for the client.

9. When you have removed one set of strips (1, 2, 3), apply the second set in the gaps (4, 5, 6), taking care not to overlap into areas already waxed.

10. If any patches of wax remain on the skin, roll a strip of used wax into a ball, with the hair side in the middle, and gently roll it over the remaining wax to remove it

11. Do not re-apply wax over already waxed areas. Tweeze any hairs that were missed, although with practice and care this should not happen.

12. When the whole area has been waxed, soothe the area with after-wax lotion.

13. Take extra care if small blood spots appear and ensure that any contaminated waste is disposed of appropriately.

14. Remember to turn off your wax heater.

15. Update your client's record card with all the details of the treatment, any contra-actions/reactions and home care advice.

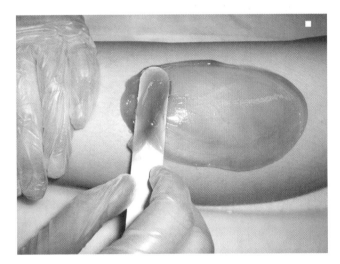

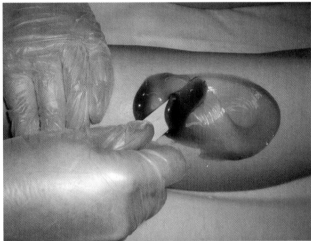

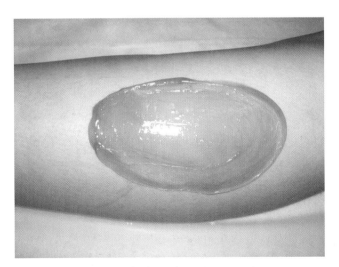

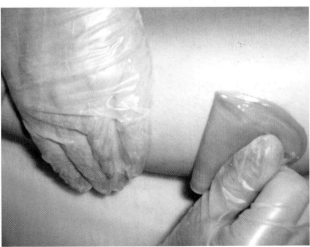

Cool wax treatments

Cool wax is sometimes called warm wax treatment, as the wax is warmed, though not to the same temperature as hot wax. Modern materials can often be used at lower temperatures, although roll-on applicators (see below) can be used at higher temperatures to treat coarser hairs.

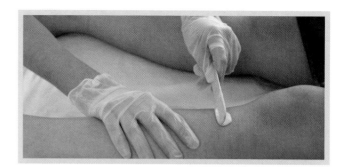

1. Heat the wax to its working temperature (approximately 43°C, but always following the manufacturer's instructions).

2. After wiping with sanitiser or pre wax lotion/gel do not apply anything else to the skin, as this will stop the wax from adhering properly.

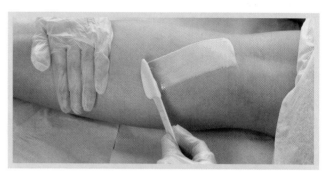

3. After testing the temperature on the therapist's wrist first and the client's wrist or ankle, apply the wax as thinly and evenly as possible to the whole area to be waxed in the direction of the hair growth, holding the spatula at right angles to the skin to ensure that the wax drips from the top to the bottom of the spatula. Use a new spatula for each new area treated unless blood spots occur in which case a new spatula should be used for each application of wax to ensure the wax pot does not become contaminated.

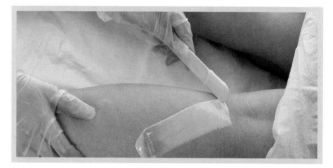

4. Place a muslin strip down firmly so it bonds with the wax, then pull pack against the direction of the hair growth in one movement, holding the skin taut with your other hand. Do not lift up and away from the skin, but parallel to it.

5. You can re-use the same strip until it is not longer effective in removing the hairs, then dispose of it safely and use a new one. However, if blood spots appear in the area, new strips must be used each time.

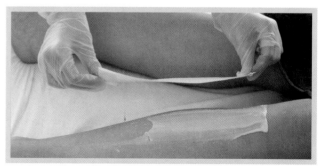

6. If all the hairs have not been removed, cool wax may be reapplied once only.

7. Any stray hairs should be tweezed out.

8. Take extra care if small blood spots appear and ensure that any contaminated waste is disposed of appropriately.

9. Remove any final traces of wax by applying an after-treatment lotion, gel or oil.

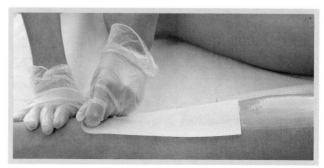

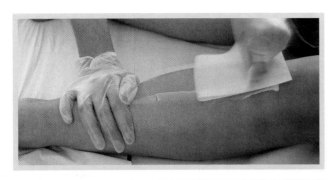

10. Remember to turn off your wax heater.

11. Dispose of all contaminated waste appropriately.

12. Update your client's record card with all the details of the treatment, any reactions and home care advice.

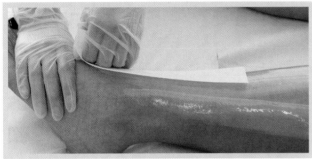

Roll-on applicators

Roll-on applicators come in a self-contained set with pre-filled applicators and their own heater. They are easy to use, with hygienic detachable, easily cleaned or disposable heads. They generally cause little discomfort to the client and are less messy than spatula methods, although their principle is the same.

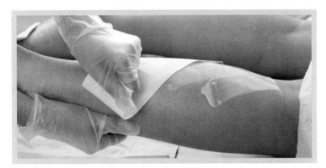

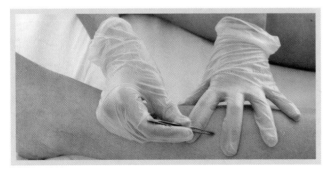

Ingrowing hairs

Ingrowing hairs usually occur when the opening of the hair follicle has become blocked and the hair starts to grow back in on itself. It can be caused by:

☐ overgrowth of the stratum corneum

☐ dry skin blocking the pores

☐ lack of moisture

☐ shaving

☐ hair breaking off during waxing

☐ poor waxing technique

☐ infrequent exfoliation

☐ inadequate care after depilatory treatments.

Regular exfoliating and moisturising can prevent ingrowing hairs.

Treating specific areas of the body

In addition to the general application methods for each treatment, specific parts of the body need to be treated in different ways.

Legs

1. Treat the front of the legs first; your client can be lying down or semi-reclined.

2. Keep the leg in a flat position for treating the front of the leg.

3. Support and tighten the skin on the thigh area when applying and removing wax.

4. Turn your client onto their front for treating the backs of the legs.

5. Be extra careful about the varying direction of hair growth on the back of the legs.

6. Do not apply wax over the back of the knee.

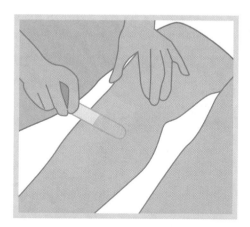

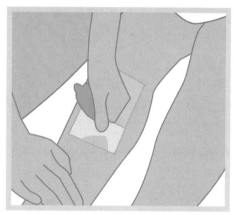

Bikini line

1. Your client should be lying down or in a semi-reclined position with their leg bent in a 'figure four' position (the tree position) and supported with a cushion.

2. You could advise your client to wear the relevant swimwear to be certain of the amount of depilation. Use tissues to protect your client's clothes.

3. If necessary, trim hairs on the first visit, to reduce length and prevent discomfort, as hairs in this area tend to be coarser and stronger. Regular waxing may reduce the coarseness of the hairs.

4. Ask the client to stretch the skin taut whilst you apply the wax in small amounts according to the direction of hair growth. You may need to use a smaller spatula.

5. Remove using smaller muslin or paper strips already cut and prepared for this area

6. Blood spots and bruising may appear in this sensitive area particularly on a first treatment.

7. If blood spots occur take extra care, and ensure that any contaminated waste is disposed of appropriately, in a plastic bag in a separate (chemical) bin.

8. When the area has been covered, tweeze out any stray hairs and wipe over with antiseptic wipes and a soothing lotion.

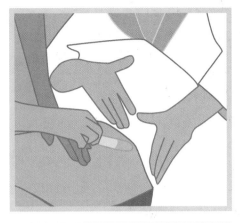

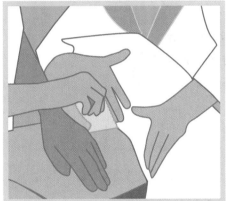

Arms

1. Bend the arms when waxing above the elbow.

2. Generally, cool wax treatment using smaller muslin/paper strips is recommended.

3. Hair growth is generally in one direction.

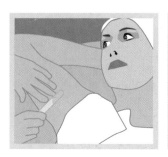
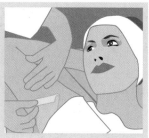

Underarms

1. Position your client comfortably, flat or semi reclined, with the arm to be treated raised behind the head.

2. Protect your client's clothing with tissues.

3. Make sure the skin is stretched taut (your client may help with their other hand).

4. Trim the hairs first if necessary.

5. Hair may grow in different directions, so check it carefully before applying the wax in small amounts or strips, working from the outside first using a small spatula.

6. Blood spots may appear in this sensitive area particularly on a first treatment.

7. If blood spots occur take extra care, and ensure that any contaminated waste is disposed of appropriately,

Lips and chin

1. Your client should be lying down.

2. Remove all traces of make-up first.

3. Gently tilt your client's head back to make the chin taut when waxing.

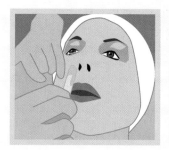
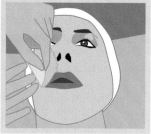

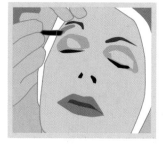
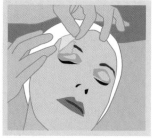

Eyebrows

See the chapter on eyebrow shaping. This treatment must be performed with great caution as the skin of the eyebrows is so fine and sensitive.

1. Your client should be lying down with eyes closed.

2. Do not use hot wax in this sensitive area.

3. Protect the hairs not to be waxed with petroleum jelly.

4. Apply the wax carefully with an orange wood stick, noting the direction of growth

Acceptable time limits

The industry standards for acceptable time limits for depilatory treatments are:

- [ ] full leg – 40 minutes
- [ ] half leg – 20 minutes
- [ ] bikini and underarms – 15 minutes
- [ ] lip and chin – 5 minutes.

However, because of variation from client to client, timings are not cut and dried, and depend on the area and density of the hair growth.

Client record card

For all treatments, you must remember to complete the client record card, noting the treatments given, products used and any contraindications, reactions and any home care advice you have given your client.

Home-care advice

As the stratum corneum has been removed during the depilatory treatment the skin will be sensitive therefore you should advise your client that for 24 to 48 hours they must:

- [ ] only wash or shower in lukewarm water
- [ ] not use exfoliators for 2–3 days depending on the skin's reaction
- [ ] use soothing after-wax gels, lotions or oils to moisturise the skin
- [ ] not use soap, deodorant or perfumed products
- [ ] not use make-up or self-tanning preparations in the area waxed
- [ ] not wear tight-fitting clothes
- [ ] not be exposed to ultra-violet light (no sunbathing or use of sunbeds)
- [ ] not have a heat treatment
- [ ] not have a stimulating treatment in the area waxed.

Giving your client an advice sheet would help to remind them of the after-care advice.

ENDPOINTS

By the end of this topic, you should understand:

- [ ] how to prepare for depilation treatments
- [ ] hot wax treatments
- [ ] cool wax
- [ ] how to deal with ingrowing hairs
- [ ] how to treat specific areas of the body
- [ ] acceptable time limits for depilation treatments
- [ ] the importance of maintaining the client record card
- [ ] home-care advice for depilation treatments.

Chapter 7:
Cosmetic science

In this chapter we'll be looking at:

introduction

Advances in beauty therapy have both driven, and been driven by, developments in cosmetic science.

The science of cosmetics has provided new techniques in response to demand from clients and therapists, and therapists have developed new techniques for their clients based on advances in cosmetic science.

Topic 1: The functions of cosmetic ingredients

The basic component of most cosmetics is an emulsion of oil-in-water, or water-in-oil, in which one component is dispersed as small (0.1μm to 50μm) droplets in the other. The balance chosen will depend on the strength of emollient properties required from a product. The size of the suspended droplets can vary, and the emulsion will become effectively transparent if their diameter is less than about 0.05μm. Most emulsions consist of two components, but it is possible to create more complex emulsions with, for example, water dispersed in the oil phas--e of an oil-in-water emulsion, to create a water-in-oil-in-water emulsion.

An emulsion starts as two liquids that are not soluble in each other, such as oil and water.

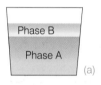

Phase B

Phase A

(a)

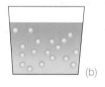

(b)

(c)

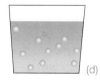

(d)

These can form an oil in water (oiw) emulsion…

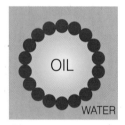

Oil in water emulsion

…or a water in oil (wio) emulsion.

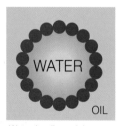

Water in oil emulsion

The micelles that form the emulsion can take several forms…

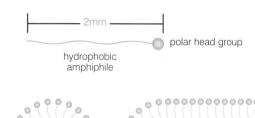

2mm

polar head group

hydrophobic amphiphile

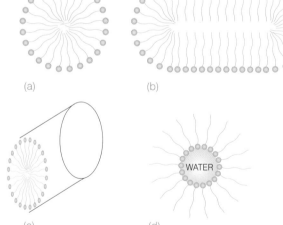

(a)

(b)

(c)

(d)

FORM OF AN AMPHIPHILE AND SEVERAL FORMS OF MICELLE: (a) SPHERICAL, (b) DISK, (c) ROD, AND (d) REVERSED.

Emulsions can break down over time, and separate into their components. If this happens the emulsion will not only appear unpleasant, but will not work as intended. To prevent this, surfactants, hydrocolloids, or fine powders are added to the emulsion. This must be done with caution, as to add too much would create an emulsion that is too stable, and does not break down fast enough when applied to the skin.

A stable cosmetic is good, but it must also be of the correct consistency for easy, even and effective application, and thickening agents may have to be added to ensure that it is not too fluid. A variety of thickening agents may be used:

Electrolytes such as:

☐ sodium chloride, which thickens by increasing the size of the surfactant micelles

☐ polymeric thickeners like polyacrylates, polyurethanes and polyamides or the polysaccharide carboxymethylcellulose work by chain entanglement

☐ gums like xanthan, guar, arabic and carrageenan

☐ inorganic compounds such as silicates and clays.

Regardless of the intended use of the cosmetic, a limited range of components are added to the basic emulsion:

☐ active ingredients

☐ colours

☐ fragrances

☐ preservatives

☐ thickeners

☐ water

☐ surfactants.

The functions of active ingredients

All the active ingredients added to cosmetics perform a function essential to the efficacy of the product, but the range of active ingredients used includes:

☐ **antioxidants** to combat free radicals in the environment, and so prevent much of the damage they do skin through oxidation and subsequent deterioration of skin cells

☐ **binding agents** to hold products together and prevent the water and lipid components from separating

☐ **emollients** to smooth and soften the skin

☐ **emulsions** – to smooth the blend of oil and water that provide a base for the product

☐ **humectants** that attract water, usually out of the air. they are effective moisturisers

☐ **lubricants** to reduce friction, making skin smoother to the touch

☐ **preservatives**, added in order to kill bacteria, yeasts, moulds and fungi that would otherwise cause the product to decay

☐ **solvents**, such as alcohol or water, used so that other ingredients can be dissolved in them

☐ **surfactants**, used because they make the product spread more easily on the skin.

ENDPOINTS
By the time you have finished this topic, you should understand:

☐ the functions of cosmetic ingredients, including the nature of an emulsion and the different main active ingredients.

Topic 2: The main mask ingredients

Clay-based masks are prepared by mixing the dry powder with a variety of active ingredients to form a smooth, easy-to-apply paste. Distilled (purified) water may be added to dilute the paste if a more liquid consistency is desired, or for hypersensitive skins.

Clay masks can be individually mixed to benefit a range of skin types and requirements. Both the clays and the active ingredients have a variety of cleansing, toning, refining and stimulating effects so the constituents, and their proportions in a mask can be varied to create products with many different overall effects.

Clay ingredients and their effects

- **Calamine** – soothes inflamed skin and reduces vascularity; suitable for sensitive skin

- **Kaolin** – deep cleanses, removes impurities, stimulates circulation, helps desquamation and improves skin function, tightening the pores. Suitable for oily, congested skin

- **Magnesium carbonate** – mildly astringent, refines skin with open pores, stimulates to tighten and firm skin; suitable for young skin, or mixed with calamine for dryer, more sensitive skins

- **Fuller's earth** – fast, strong action on blood circulation, excellent desquamation and deep cleansing; ideal for oily, congested skin, not suitable for sensitive skin

- **Flowers of sulphur** – very strong drawing, drying effect, dissolves surface dead skin cells, generally added to fuller's earth for use on extremely oily skin

Active ingredients and their effects

These should be matched to the clays for the appropriate skin type. While it is not itself an active ingredient, distilled water forms a perfect carrier for active ingredients, and its purity makes it less likely to irritate a sensitive skin. Active ingredients include:

- **Rosewater** – mildly toning effect, for mature, dry and sensitive skins

- **Orange flower water** – mildly toning effect, suitable for all skin types

- **Witch hazel** – an astringent, drying and stimulating effect, for oily skin

- **Glycerine** – soothing and moisturising, for dry and dehydrated skin, a humectant which helps keep mask soft

- **Almond oil** – slightly stimulating and nourishing, helps hydration of dry skin.

ENDPOINTS

By the time you have finished this topic, you should understand:

- the main mask ingredients, both clay and active, their uses and effects.

Topic 3: Natural ingredients

Natural ingredients are valuable components of modern cosmetic products. Natural ingredients are simple but effective, as plant enzymes can trigger reactions even in the deepest layers of the skin's cells. These ingredients may come from:

- ☐ fruit
- ☐ plants
- ☐ herbs
- ☐ natural products, e.g. eggs, yoghurts and honey.

Natural ingredients and their effects

Natural ingredients have a variety of cosmetic uses and effects, as we saw earlier.

- ☐ **Aloe** – soothing/calming for sensitive skins, very beneficial for sunburn
- ☐ **Avocado** – very gentle on skin, with natural vitamins and minerals; its natural oil is beneficial for dry, mature or sensitive skins
- ☐ **Banana** – contains potassium, calcium, phosphates and vitamins; good for dry and sensitive skins
- ☐ **Carrots** – stimulates cell regeneration
- ☐ **Cucumber** – cooling effect, helps to soothe tired eyes; good for oily skins; toning and refining
- ☐ **Egg white** – has a toning and tightening effect, best for young or oily skin types;
- ☐ **Egg yolk** – nourishes the skin; good for dry skins
- ☐ **Herbs** – tone, stimulate, balance and regenerate; good for all skin types.
- ☐ **Honey** – used to remove impurities and dead skin cells; lightens and hydrates skin, delaying formation of lines; mature or sensitive skins
- ☐ **Kiwi** – moisturising for dry, dehydrated skins and contains vitamin C

- ☐ **Lemon juice** – very stimulating; good for oily skin
- ☐ **Marine products** – hydrate and stabilise the skin
- ☐ **Milk** – good base for natural masks
- ☐ **Natural yoghurt** – makes a good base for masks
- ☐ **Oatmeal** – good for desquamation
- ☐ **Pear** – soft fruit, see below
- ☐ **Soft fruits**, such as strawberries, have an acid reaction on skin (can be mixed with yoghurt, cream or egg white to lessen acidic reaction), correct the pH balance of dry skin and increase moisture level
- ☐ **Teabags** – soothing for the eyes, use cold
- ☐ **Wheatgerm** – contains vitamin E good for dry, mature skins

The inclusion of some natural products in cosmetics can raise issues for both the cosmetic scientist/manufacturer and the beauty therapist. Some natural ingredients are perishable, and may require preparation at the time of use, or the addition of preservatives or anti-oxidants to prevent them

THE ART AND SCIENCE OF BEAUTY THERAPY

decaying or becoming ineffective. Some natural ingredients may also be contra-indicated for some clients, and so the therapist should:

☐ ensure they understand the nature of the ingredients in any cosmetic product and their potential side-effects

☐ perform any necessary preliminary sensitivity tests

☐ check the client's record card for indications of sensitivity to a product.

For more information on contra-indications and record-keeping, see Chapter 1.

Safety
Always check for allergies if using a product with natural ingredients. Always ensure that natural ingredients are within their expiry date, or freshly prepared.

ENDPOINTS
By the time you have finished this topic, you should understand:

☐ the sources and uses of natural ingredients

☐ the importance of record-keeping in relation to the use of natural ingredients.

Topic 4: Cosmetic ingredients

As therapists, we have a professional responsibility and legal duty to use appropriate products for our clients. Part of this entails knowing about the ingredients in the products we use, so that we, and our clients have the most beneficial outcomes. To do this, we need to know what the ingredients in the products we use are for, and what their effects can be.

Legislation

The Cosmetic Products (Safety) Regulations 2004 came in to force on 11th September 2004, and defines a cosmetic product as being:

"Any substance or preparation placed in contact with any part of the external surfaces of the human body (that is to say, the epidermis hair system, nails and external genital organs), or with the teeth and the mucous membranes of the oral cavity, with a view exclusively or mainly to cleaning them, perfuming them, changing their appearance, protecting them, keeping them in good condition or correcting body odours, except where such cleaning, perfuming, protecting, changing, keeping, or correcting is wholly for the purpose of treating or preventing disease."

Note that products used solely as medicines are not covered by these Regulations. The main provisions of the regulations are that:

☐ it is an offence to supply cosmetic products that are liable to cause damage to human health when applied under normal conditions of use, or reasonably foreseeable conditions of use

☐ many substances are either prohibited or restricted for use in cosmetic products, although some substances are not subject to the Regulations if the product was supplied before 24th September 2005

☐ certain labeling standards are required.

Marking and labeling of cosmetics
Cosmetic products must be labeled with their ingredients, name and address of manufacturer, batch code and durability (or use-by date). All the information must be visible, indelible, easily legible, and in English.

Ingredients
The packaging of the product must carry a list of ingredients, headed 'Ingredients', in descending order of weight. Some things do not need to appear in this list, such as:

☐ impurities in the raw materials

☐ materials used in the preparation of, but not present in, the final product

☐ materials used as solvents or carriers for perfumes and aromatic compositions.

Perfume and aromatic compositions and their raw materials may be referred to as 'perfume' or 'aroma'. Ingredients that make up less than 1% of the product may be listed in any order after those that make up 1% or more, and colours may be listed in any order after the other ingredients. So that ingredients can be identified easily by therapists and their clients across the EU, the ingredient names listed should be those listed in the International Nomenclature of Cosmetic Ingredients (INCI). If the INCI list does not contain an approved name for the ingredient, then an alternative is to use the:

☐ chemical name

☐ CTFA name

☐ European Pharmacopoeia name

- International Non-proprietary Name (INN), as recommended by the World Health Organisation
- EINECS identification
- IUPAC or CAS identification
- colour index number.

Name and address

The labeling must give the name and address of the manufacturer or supplier of the product.

Function

If it is not obvious from the design and packaging what the product is for, it must be written on the label.

Batch code

A batch code provides a method of identifying the production batch from which the particular sample of product came in case of any problems. This is normally a code or date.

Durability

The ingredients (particularly those of a natural origin) in some cosmetic products can deteriorate as they age, and some products will contain preservatives or stabilisers to ameliorate this. If, however, a cosmetic product is likely, within 30 months of the date of manufacture, to deteriorate to the extent that it is liable to cause damage to human health, it must be marked with an appropriate 'Best Before' date and details of any storage precautions needed to meet that date. Since 2005, products should be labeled with the symbol below, and an indication of their life after opening. Generally speaking, cosmetic preparations have a life of two years unopened and six months once opened.

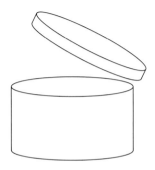

Common cosmetic ingredients

Use of the common INCI names for cosmetic ingredients makes it possible to identify the substances by using a unique name, with the result that therapists and consumers can easily identify ingredients that they have been advised to avoid (for example because of allergies).

The list of ingredients on some cosmetics can be very long. In order to know which product to use for your client, and which may be contraindicated, it is essential to know the main characteristics of those ingredients. Here is a list (in alphabetical order) of some of the more common ingredients, with their INCI names:

INCI name	Description	Use
Acetone	Acetone	A solvent, most commonly found as nail varnish remover. Can dry or irritate skin
Alcohol	Ethanol	Used as a vehicle for cosmetic ingredients, as it evaporates rapidly on the skin, and may have bactericidal properties
Algae	Algae/seaweed extract	An emollient, restoring moisture content to skin; claimed to have antioxidant properties
Alkanna Tinctoria extract	Alkanet root extract	Tonic
Aloe Barbadensis extract	Aloe Vera juice	Emollient
Sodium Alum	Alum, Aluminium sodium bis(sulphate)	An astringent used in styptic (haemostatic) sticks to stem bleeding
Prunus Armeniaca (Apricot) seed powder	Powder ground from the seeds of the apricot, Prunus armeniaca, Rosaceae	Abrasive

Arnica montana extract	Arnica	Tonic/emollient/antidandruff/ antimicrobial/helps bruising
Ascorbic acid	Ascorbic acid (vitamin C)	An antioxidant and skin-lightener
Ascorbyl palmitate	Ascorbyl palmitate (vitamin C ester)	A fat and water soluble antioxidant used in topical products and as an alternative form of Vitamin C
Melissa Officinalis (Lemon Balm) extract	Balm Mint	Soothing/astringent/masking
Cera alba	Beeswax	Used as a barrier and water retainer in topical cosmetics
Aluminium Silicate	Bentonite clay	Cosmetic colourant
Boric acid	Boric acid	Antimicrobial
Caffeine	Caffeine	Skin conditioning, used to alleviate puffiness under eyes.
Calendula Officinalis	Calendula	Emollient flower extract
Camphor	Camphor	Denaturant, plasticiser, cooling agent used to help alleviate itching and irritation in many skin care and medicated products.
Candelilla sera	The candelilla wax obtained from Euphorbia cerifera, Euphorbiaceae	Emollient/film forming used in lipstick

Carbomer	Carbomers (934, 940, 941, 980, 981)	Stabilises and thickens products.
Carmine	Carmine	A red pigment that can cause irritation used in eyeshadows and lipsticks to produce red/rust shades
Cera Carnauba	Carnauba wax. The wax derived from Copernicia cerifera, Arecaceae	Emollient/film forming. Used in lipsticks
Cellulose	Cellulose	The basic structural matter in plants, used to thicken products or to stabilise suspensions
Ceramide	Ceramides	An epidermal hydrating agent, hair and skin conditioning
Ceteareth	Ceteareth	A lubricant made from a combination of cetearyl and stearyl alcohols
Cetyl Alcohol	Cetyl Alcohol	Used to help form oil/water emulsions and as a lubricant
Anthemis Nobilis extract	Chamomile Roman. An extract of the flowers of the chamomile, Anthemis nobilis, Compositae	Tonic/skin conditioning
CI 75810	Chlorophyll	Cosmetic colourant
Cinnamomum Cassia	Cinnamomum Cassia is a plant material derived from the dried bark of the cinnamon, Cinnamomum cassia, Lauraceae.	Oral care/face masks/hair conditioning
Citric Acid	Citric Acid	Buffering/chelating

Theobroma Cacao butter	Cocoa butter. Theobroma Cacao Butter is a yellowish white solid material obtained from the roasted seeds of Theobroma cacao, Sterculiaceae	Emollient
Collagen	Collagen. A fibrous protein comprising one third of the total protein in mammals.It is a polypeptide containing three peptide chains and rich in proline and hydroxyproline.	Makes up the main supporting fibres of the skin, and is used topically to hydrate and moisturise
Symphytum Officinale extract	Comfrey. Symphytum Officinale Extract is an extract of the rhizomes and roots of the comfrey, Symphytum officinale,Boraginaceae	Soothing/antidandruff
Cyclomethicone	Cyclomethicone	Silicone compounds that give a smooth texture to products also antistatic/emollient/humectant/ solvent/viscosity controlling/hair conditioning
Dimethicone	Dimethicone	Antifoaming/emollient
Alcohol denatured	Ethanol denatured in accordance with Customs and Excise regulations	Solvent
Elastin	Elastin	In the skin, elastin provides elasticicity and support in topical cosmetics it is used to aid the appearance of wrinkles and reduce moisture loss
EDTA	Ethylenediaminetetraacetic acid (EDTA)	Used as preservative and stabilising agent, chelating
Glycerine	Glycerol	A humectant

Glycine	Glycine	A key amino acid in collagen production. Antistatic/buffering/ skin conditioning/hair conditioning
Glycol stearate	Glycol stearate	Used to give a cosmetic an opalescent appearance and thicker consistency
Glycolic acid	Glycolic acid	An exfoliant AHA used in chemical peels, and for acne, dry skin, pores and wrinkles
Caprae Lac	Goats' milk	Skin conditioning
Palmitoyl grape seed	Grape seed, vitis vinifera, extract, reaction products with hexadecanoyl chloride	Extracts used as an antioxidant
Citrus Grandis seed extract	Grapefruit seed extract (GSE)	Skin conditioning/ astringent/tonic
Hyaluronic acid	Hyaluronic acid	A powerful hydrating agent due to the amount of water it can hold
Hydroquinone	Hydroquinone	Used as a skin-lightener
Isopropyl alcohol	Isopropyl alcohol	Used as a vehicle – antibacterial, but can dry the skin
Isopropyl isostearate	Isopropyl isostearate	An emollient used to condition and soften the skin
Isopropyl palmitate	Isopropyl palmitate	A thickening agent and emollient derived from palm or coconut oils

Isostearic acid	Isostearic acid or Isooctadecanoic acid.	A commonly used emulsifier
Simmondsia Chinensis powder	Jojoba powder (a powder of the ground seeds of the jojoba, Simmondsia chinensis, Buxaceae)	Skin conditioning
Kaolin	Kaolin (China clay or aluminium silicate)	Used as an absorbent
Kojic acid	Kojic acid (5-hydroxy-2-hydroxymethyl-4-pyrone)	Used as a skin lightener, but may have a short shelf-life
Lanolin	Lanolin. Fat-like substance derived from sheep wool. Contains a complex combination of esters and polyesters, consisting chiefly of cholesteryl and isocholesteryl esters of the higher fatty acids.	An animal-derived emollient and moisturiser – could cause contact dermatitis
Lecithin	Lecithin	Helps hydrate skin and improves product texture
Lactuca Scariola extract	Lettuce extract	Soothing/refreshing
Glycyrrhiza Glabra extract	Licorice extract	An extract of the roots of the licorice, Glycyrrhiza glabra, Leguminosae, used as a skin lightening ingredient
Linoleic acid	Linoleic acid (vitamin F)	Used in emulsions and to hydrate skin
Lysine	Lysine	A skin-conditioning amino acid

Menthol	Mentholum	Denaturant/soothing/refreshing/masking
Avena Sativa flour	Oat flour	Abrasive/absorbent/viscosity controlling
Benzophenone-3	Oxybenzone	A UVA-absorbing ingredient in sunscreens
Panthenol	Panthenol (vitamin B5)	A humectant
Petrolatum	Petroleum jelly	Used as a base but, whilst good for sensitive skin, may cause pores to clog
Solanum Tuberosum starch	Potato starch	Has a slight tightening effect on the skin
Proline	Proline	An key amino acid in collagen production
Propylene glycol	Propylene glycol	Used as a basis for cosmetic solutions. It has excellent hydration qualities but can be contraindicated for dermatitis
Retinol	Retinol	A fat-soluble Vitamin A derivative. Rejuvenating
Retinyl Palmitate	Retinyl Palmitate	The ester formed from retinol and palmitic acid. Helps smooth fine lines
Oryza Sativa (Rice)	Oryza Sativa Extract is an extract of the grains of rice, Oryza sativa, Gramineae	Skin conditioning/hair conditioning/bulking/absorbent/abrasive
Salicylic acid	Salicylic (beta-hydroxy) acid	Used in chemical peels. An exfoliant that can reduce the appearance of fine lines and counter oiliness and acne

Butyrospermum Parkii butter	Shea butter. Butyrospermum Parkii Butter is the fat obtained from the fruit of the karite tree, Butyrospernum parkii, Sapotaceae	Skin conditioning/emollient
Silicone	Silicone	Used to protect and give a sheen to skin
Silica	Silica, Silicon dioxide.	A highly oil absorbent mineral, also abrasive/absorbent/ opacifying/viscosity controlling/anticaking/bulking
Sodium stearoyl, Hydrolyzed silk	Silk protein – Hydrolysed silk protein, N-octanoyl derivatives, sodium salts	An ingredient used in eye rejuvenation creams to prevent dehydration
Sodium Bicarbonate	Sodium Bicarbonate	Commonly known as baking soda, Sodium Bicarbonate is used to reduce acidity and hence irritation
Sodium Borate	Sodium Borate	A preservative, but can cause irritation
Sodium Chloride	Sodium Chloride	Used for viscosity control/bulking
Sorbic acid	Sorbic acid	A preservative used to prevent growth of yeasts in cosmetics
Sorbitan Stearate	Sorbitan monostearate	Emulsifier
Sorbitol	Sorbitol	A derivative of sugar used to hydrate the skin, which it does by attracting and holding water. If, however, the air is drier than the skin, it will attempt to absorb water from the skin, causing dehydration.

Stearic Acid	Stearic Acid	An essential fatty acid used to make soap – may irritate
Sulfur	Sulphur	Used as topical bactericide in soaps, shampoos, etc. to combat acne and similar conditions
Titanium dioxide	Titanium dioxide	Opacifies, used to block UVA and UVB
Solanum Lycopersicum juice	Tomato juice	Skin conditioner
Triclosan	Triclosan	A hypoallergenic preservative
Tyrosine	Tyrosine	An amino acid that stimulates collagen production and melanin formation
Tocopherol	Vitamin E	A moisturiser and antioxidant used in cosmetics to protect the skin from the effects of UV radiation
Tocopheryl Acetate	Vitamin E Acetate	Antioxidant
Aqua	Water	The most common main ingredient of skin care products
Tritcum Vulgare Germ	Wheat Germ	Skin protecting/skin conditioning
Xanthan gum	Xanthan gum	Used as a thickening agent

ENDPOINTS

By the time you have finished this topic, you should understand:

☐ the legal definition of cosmetic ingredients and the requirements regarding their labeling, naming and storage.

Chapter 8: The science of electrical treatments

In this chapter we'll be looking at:

introduction

As beauty therapists we are aiming to improve the overall condition of the skin. This sometimes requires a deeper, more intense treatment, which may require the use of electrical equipment.

Effective, professional and safe practice requires us to understand something of the interactions and techniques we are employing, together with their effects and implications for the client and therapist.

Topic 1:
The structure of the atom

The world around us (and including us) us is made up of a myriad of tiny particles, called atoms. These atoms are of a number of different types, or elements, such as carbon, iron, oxygen or hydrogen. The existence of atoms as one of the smallest building blocks of the physical world was first suggested by the ancient Greek, Democritus, but really became an accepted model when restated by Dalton in the 19th century.

An understanding of atoms, their structure and behaviour permits an understanding of many of the physical effects that we use or harness as beauty therapists. Atoms, combined together through chemical reactions to form molecules, make up the world around us, the cosmetic products we use and even our clients and ourselves.

The atom

Just as we are made of many molecules, and molecules are made of a number of atoms, atoms themselves are made up of a number of smaller sub-atomic particles, called protons, neutrons and electrons.

The atoms of different elements are constructed of different numbers of these particles and hence have different atomic weights. These are expressed relative to the mass of a carbon atom, which is set at 12. On this scale, a hydrogen atom (the lightest atom) has a mass of 1.

Smaller and smaller

Everything is composed of tiny particles called atoms, and they themselves are composed of smaller sub-atomic particles, called protons, neutrons and electrons.

Sub-atomic particles

The protons and neutrons (which have similar masses very close to 1) within an atom form a nucleus at its centre, about which the electrons (which have a relatively tiny mass) orbit. A hydrogen atom, which has a mass of 1, will have one proton in its nucleus, with a single electron orbiting it.

The three particles vary in other ways besides their mass. Neutrons, as their name implies, are electrically neutral. Protons, on the other hand, have a positive electrical charge. Each electron in the atom has a negative electrical charge of the same size as the positive charge on a proton. The positively charged protons, and negatively charged electrons are attracted together. In an atom, there are the same number of protons and electrons, leaving atoms electrically neutral overall.

Ions

If an atom loses or gains electrons, so that it no longer has an equal number of electrons and protons, then its overall electrical charge will no longer be zero and, in this state, it is called an ion. If it has gained electrons it will have become negatively charged overall, and is known as an anion, and if it has lost electrons (becoming positively charged), it will be known as a cation.

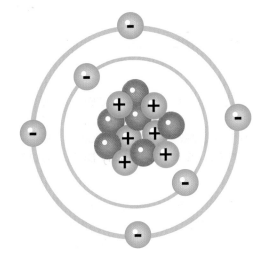

CARBON ATOM

	proton	=	6
-	electron	=	6
	neutron	=	6

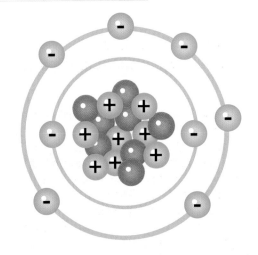

OXYGEN

	proton	=	8
-	electron	=	8
	neutron	=	8

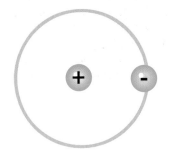

HYDROGEN

	proton	=	1
-	electron	=	1
	neutron	=	0

ENDPOINTS
By the end of this topic, you should understand:

☐   the structure of the atom.

247

Topic 2: Electricity

We need power to drive the appliances and tools we use in beauty therapy, and electricity, almost always supplied through the mains, is the most common source of power for our equipment and plays a direct part in some of the treatments we provide.

The measurement of electricity

An electrical current (measured in Amperes, or Amps, symbol A) is a flow of electrons through a conductor such as a wire. This flow of electrons is caused by an applied potential difference (measured in Volts, symbol V) or voltage. A simple way to think of this is as the voltage representing the pressure on the water in a hosepipe, and the current representing the flow of water through the pipe.

The voltage and current are related. For the same piece of wire, a higher voltage results in a higher current, and vice versa – much as turning up the tap to a hosepipe results in a greater flow of water through it. The relationship between voltage and current is expressed through Ohm's law, which introduces another factor – resistance – to describe the characteristics of the conductor. To continue our hosepipe analogy, if we replace our normal hosepipe with a very narrow one, less water will flow through for the same setting on the tap. The resistance of a conductor is a measure of its resistance to current flowing through it. For the same voltage, a higher resistance allows less current to flow than a lower resistance.

Ohm's law is very simple:
Voltage = Current x Resistance or $V = I \times R$

Types of electric current

An alternating (AC) current flows in one direction, then the other, continually reversing, much as the flow of water in waves on a beach flows back and forth. A direct (DC) current flows in one direction only, as the water in a river flows in one direction only. The current that flows from a mains socket into an appliance is an alternating current – you will see the inputs to equipment marked with the voltage they accept and that it is AC.

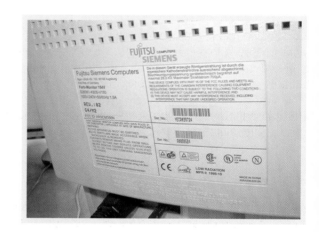

The dangers of electrical currents

Electrical currents can be dangerous if not used correctly. The electrical shock from a malfunctioning piece of salon equipment can be as lethal as a lightning strike, and so the proper selection, usage, maintenance and testing of electrical equipment is essential.

The physiological risks of electrical currents

The physical damage caused by electrical currents falls into three main areas – burns, effects on the heart and neurological system.

1. **Burns**. As the current tries to flow through the body, the resistance of the body causes tissues to heat up. This can cause severe burns deep in the body, especially at higher voltages with sources that can provide high currents.

2. **The heart**. The effect of an electrical shock on the heart can cause ventricullar fibrillation – disrupting the contraction of the muscles of the heart – which

is usually lethal. Even at a low voltage such as that supplied by the mains (240v AC), ventricular fibrillation may be induced in the heart after a fraction of a second of a current as low as a twentieth of an Ampere travelling through the chest. A higher current is needed if the voltage is DC.

3. **Effects on the neurological system**. An electric shock can affect the operation of the nervous system, affecting the heart and lungs in particular. If the shock runs through the head, a large enough current can cause unconsciousness and death.

The effects of therapeutic electrical currents on body tissues

1. Faradic treatments

Faradic treatments are used to tone muscles and firm facial contours. In a Faradic treatment a low-voltage direct current is applied under the control of the therapist, via an electrode placed on the skin on the mnotor point of the muscle that requires stimulation. This causes the muscle to contract (stimulation period) and relax (stimulation interval).

2. Galvanic treatments

Galvanic facial treatments such as desincrustination and iontophoresis employ a constant, direct low voltage current, which flows through the skin between an active electrode and an indifferent electrode. Active substances will be drawn by this current, either from the skin or into the skin. The polarity of the electrodes

is selected by the therapist depending on the polarity of the active substances.

Desincrustation is used for deep cleansing of oily skins or those prone to comedones and blemishes. An alkaline solution is placed on the skin, and the negative electrode moved over the skin. These combine to form a chemical reaction which breaks down the stearic (fatty) acid on the skin releasing blockages in the pores by softening the sebum.

Iontophoresis is used to introduce active water soluble substances into the epidermis and, through the appropriate choice of active substance, can be used for the improvement of a variety of skin types.

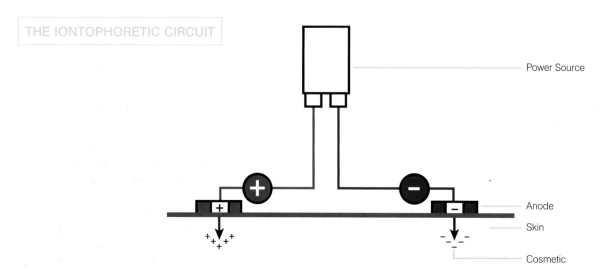

Power Source

Anode

Skin

Cosmetic

An active substance is applied to the skin. The electrode carrying the same charge as the active substance will repel the active substance into the skin The choice of treatment depends on the polarity of the active substance so it is vital the manufacturer's instructions are always adhered to – the positively charged electrode will repel a positively charged substance, and the negatively charged electrode will repel a negatively charged one.

The rate of iontophoretic transport is affected by several factors including skin pH, active ingredient concentration, current, voltage, time applied and skin resistance.

Microcurrent treatments

Microcurrent treatments use low-frequency (1 to 20 Hz) microcurrents (amounting to micro-amps) to re-educate muscle tone, shortening muscle fibres where they lack tone. The low current is undetectable to the client.

The stimulation should improve the appearance of the skin by stimulating and tightening the facial muscles and through increasing blood flow to the area. It is frequently used as an anti-ageing treatment and is often referred to as the 'face lift without the knife'.

Modified direct current

Modified direct current treatments use a varying, but still direct, current to stimulate the facial muscles.

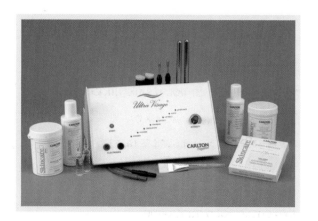

Transformers

We may sometimes need a higher or lower voltage than the 240V available from the mains supply. To achieve this, salon equipment incorporates a device called a transformer. The transformer is a device that can increase or decrease the voltage of an AC supply. It cannot change the voltage of a DC supply, nor can it affect the frequency of an AC one.

A transformer that has a higher output voltage than input voltage is called a step-up transformer, and one that has a lower output than input voltage is called a step-down transformer.

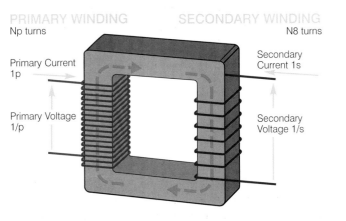

PRIMARY WINDING
Np turns

SECONDARY WINDING
N8 turns

Primary Current 1p

Secondary Current 1s

Primary Voltage 1/p

Secondary Voltage 1/s

A transformer is to be found inside the power supply of almost every piece of electrical equipment used by the therapist, where it is used to reduce the voltage of the incoming mains supply to a level more suitable for use in the equipment, machines that use an alternating current, such as high-frequency machines will also include one.

Rectifiers

We saw earlier that there are two types of current: alternating and direct. We may need to convert AC current, which is supplied in the mains supply, to DC.

To do this we use a device called a rectifier. In most cases, you will never see a rectifier – it will be a component contained within the power supply of a piece of equipment. To covert AC current to DC current, we need to stop it flowing back and forth, and to make it flow in one direction only. This is the function of the rectifier. The rectifier itself contains electronic components called diodes, which only allow current to flow in one direction – they are like doors which only open in one direction.

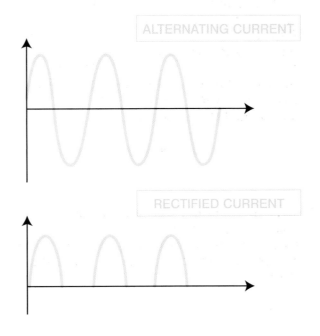

ALTERNATING CURRENT

RECTIFIED CURRENT

By the end of this topic, you should understand:

☐ the measurement of electricity

☐ the different types of current used in beauty therapy

☐ the possible risks involved

☐ the effects of currents on body tissue

☐ the function of a transformer

☐ the function of a rectifier.

Topic 3: Electromagnetic radiation and beauty therapy

Light, radio waves, ultra-violet and infra-red are all types of electromagnetic radiation. We spend our lives bathed in electromagnetic radiation from a variety of natural and artificial sources and, in our work as beauty therapists, we harness the effects of various types of electromagnetic radiation on the body in order to help our clients.

However, as anyone who has spent too long on the beach can testify, electromagnetic radiation (in this case the ultra-violet light in sunlight) can have unpleasant effects on the skin.

Professionalism, safety and efficiency therefore require that we understand the nature, behaviour and effects of the various different types of electromagnetic radiation.

The structure of the electromagnetic spectrum

The light in which we see our world is made up of a mixture of coloured light of different wavelengths – which we can see separated out into a spectrum when we see a rainbow, or look at the light reflected from the underside of a CD.

The spectrum of electromagnetic radiation runs across a range of frequencies and wavelengths, extending above and below the visible portion of the spectrum. The visible portion of the spectrum is determined by the nature of our own eyes – much as the range of sounds we can hear depends on the nature of our ears. With sound there are sounds pitched above and below the range of human senses that we cannot hear. Just as sounds range in frequency across a wide spectrum, so does electromagnetic radiation range above and below the range of our own senses, extending down in frequency from the red end of the visible part of the spectrum to infra-red radiation and then down further to radio waves, and up in frequency from the violet end of the visible spectrum into ultra-violet light, and then upwards towards X-rays, gamma-rays and cosmic rays.

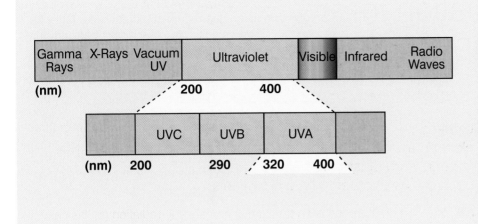

Different types of electromagnetic radiation

Radiation from the electromagnetic spectrum is all around us, from the radio waves generated by our mobile phones, to the colours of sunlight and up to and beyond the UV light from sunbeds.

The effects of electromagnetic radiation on body tissues

Just as a sound can be loud or soft, electromagnetic radiation can be more or less intense – such as from a bright or dim light.

Just as a sound can be high or low-pitched, electromagnetic radiation can be high or low-frequency. The effect a sound has on us varies with both the pitch (or frequency) and the volume (or intensity). A really high-pitched whining sound might make our teeth stand on edge, and a very low frequency sound from something like ferry-boat engines can make our stomachs churn. Sound of intense volume endured night after night when clubbing can physically damage our ears.

Just as sound waves can physically affect our bodies, so can electromagnetic radiation. Just as the effects of sound waves on our body depend on the frequency, intensity and length of exposure to the sound, so do the effects of electromagnetic radiation.

In beauty therapy, we make use of electromagnetic radiation in the infra-red region of the spectrum (with a wavelength of 4000 to 1000 nm) and in the ultra-violet region (from around 100 nm to 400 nm).

Infra-red radiation in beauty therapy

Beauty therapy makes use of two types:

1. Infra-red (4000 nm wavelength)
2. Radiant heat (1000 nm).

An infra-red lamp uses an electrical filament to heat a clay element inside a focusing reflector until it emits radiation. The radiation is invisible, and the clay element does not glow when hot. The lamp will therefore be fitted with a guard to protect against touching the hot element.

Infra-red lamps are used for heating the skin (which must be clean and grease-free) before treatment, and exposures should not last longer than 10 minutes to prevent burning of the skin. The rays themselves do not penetrate deeply into the skin, but generate heat that causes vasodilation and increases blood and lymph flow. The radiation can damage the eye, causing cataracts, and so goggles should be worn, or eyes covered with damp cotton wool pads.

Lamps that produce radiant heat are now far more common in salon use. The lamp looks like a large light bulb, and contains a filament that emits small amounts of visible and ultra-violet light in addition to infra-red heat. This is filtered by the characteristic red glass filter on the end of the lamp to ensure that no UV light reaches the client, only red and IR light.

Radiant heat lamps warm up more quickly than infra-red lamps, but still become very hot in use. The lamp must not be allowed to touch and burn the skin, and care should be taken not to knock the lamp or splash fluids on it when it is hot, as this may cause it to shatter.

Because of the vasodilatory effect of infra-red, it is contraindicated for clients with conditions such as broken capillaries and high colour or hyper-sensitive skins.

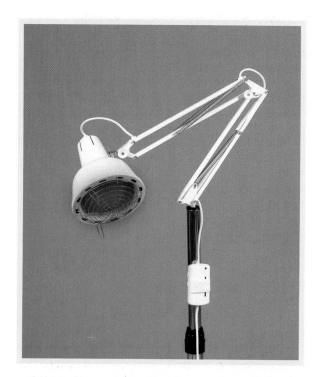

Ultra-violet radiation in beauty therapy

As well as using infra-red radiation in beauty therapy, we use electromagnetic radiation from beyond the other end of the visible spectrum. This is ultra-violet (or UV) light, and is an invisible part of the spectrum that is higher in frequency than the violet end of the visible spectrum. UV light is classified into three types based on its wavelength (these figures may vary slightly):

1. UVA 320 to 400 nanometres

2. UVB 290 to 320 nanometres

3. UVC 100 to 290 nanometres.

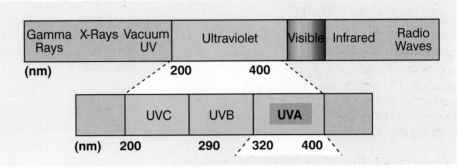

The different types of UV light penetrate to different depths in the skin, reaching different layers as they do so.

PENETRATION OF DIFFERENT UV WAVELENGTHS

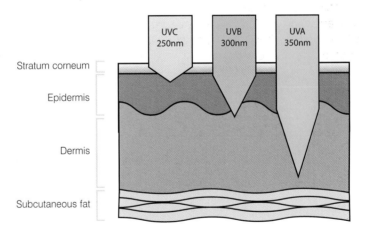

Ultraviolet light makes up about 5% of the radiation from the sun. In therapeutic use, it is generated in UV lamps containing mercury vapour. This may be at low pressure in the familiar tubes (LPMV), or high pressure (HPMV) in bulb-shaped lamps.

LPMV tubes produced almost entirely UVA light, with less than 1% UVB and almost no UVC. HPMV tubes produce all types of UV light, but reduce UVB and UVC levels to those of LPMV tubes by use of a filter that absorbs the unwanted radiation.

UV light is used in sunbeds, canopies and cubicles to produce a cosmetic tan. The tanning response, which is due to the activity of melanocytes in the epidermis and oxidation and redistribution of existing melanin, begins during the exposure to UV radiation, is highest immediately after the treatment finishes, and will fade within an hour after exposure. The tanning effect will not provide protection for the skin against natural UV radiation. Tanning of any form is detrimental to all skin types, producing premature ageing, sun damage and possible skin cancers.

The inverse square law

The closer we are to a heater, the hotter it feels, the closer we are to a lamp, the brighter it appears. The intensity of the radiation we feel from the source increases as we move closer to it, and reduces as we move further away. The radiation from a source (lamp, UV tube, etc.) escapes in all directions, spreading out as it does so. As you can see in the diagram, the amount of radiation that passes through an area of one square centimetre at a distance of one metre is the same as that passing through an area of four square centimetres at a distance of two metres. So the energy per square centimetre (or intensity) is reduced by a factor of four if the distance doubles.

Why is the inverse square law important to therapists?

As the intensity reduces by a factor of four if you double the distance, this means that if you halve the distance between a client and a lamp you quadruple the intensity of the radiation on their skin. For the therapist, this is critically important when calculating safe and effective exposure times for their clients.

INTENSITY VS DISTANCE GRAPH

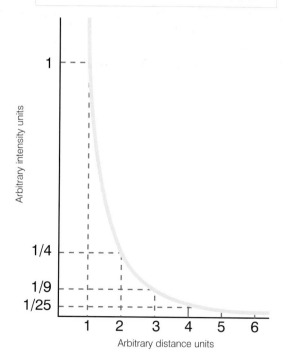

THE INVERSE SQUARE LAW DIAGRAM

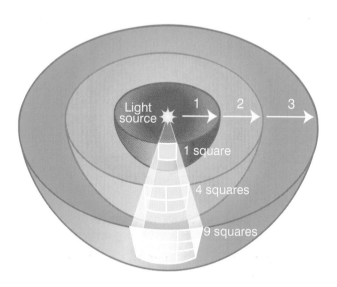

The intensity of the radiation is inversely proportional to the square of the distance from the source of the radiation – hence the name inverse square law.

The link between distance, intensity and exposure times

The intensity of rays varies inversely with the square of the distance from the lamp. Thus, the intensity of radiation from the same lamp at 30cm is 4 times that at 60cm and 11 times that at 1 metre, so a 1 minute exposure at 30cm distance is the equivalent of 4 mins at 60cm and approximately 11 mins at 1 metre.

Safety

Always remember that halving the distance between a client and a light source has the same effect as quadrupling the time they are exposed. Remember to base distances on the closest part of the client to the lamp.

ENDPOINTS

By the end of this topic, you should understand:

- [ ] the structure of the electromagnetic spectrum

- [ ] the effects of electromagnetic radiation on body tissues

- [ ] the uses of infra-red radiation in beauty therapy

- [ ] the uses of ultra-violet radiation in beauty therapy

- [ ] the inverse square law

- [ ] the link between distance, intensity and exposure times.

Topic 4: Electricity, safety and professionalism

Re-read Chapter 1, to remind yourself about general but essential health and safety precautions, and about your and the salon's liability when dealing with the general public. When using electrical equipment, the most important pieces of legislation are:

☐ the Health and Safety at Work Act 1974 (HASWA)

☐ the Electricity at Work Act 1992.

Health and Safety at Work Act 1974

HASWA details the duties of both employer and employee towards health, safety and welfare of employees, and health and safety in the workplace. Failure in these duties may result in criminal liability and claims for damages, as well as serious consequences for people's health.

For the employer, the duties which relate to using electrical equipment include:

☐ providing and maintaining:

– safe systems at work

– a safe work place

– safe access and exits to the work place

☐ ensuring the safe handling, use and storage of substances and equipment

☐ providing the necessary information, instruction, training and supervision for health and safety.

For the employee, these duties include:

☐ taking reasonable care of themselves, their clients or other staff for whom they are responsible

☐ not intentionally or recklessly misusing anything provided for health, safety or welfare.

The Electricity at Work Act 1992

This Act regulates the use of electrical equipment. Its regulations include:

☐ having every piece of electrical equipment tested at least once a year by a qualified electrician

☐ keeping a written record of all tests which can be inspected

☐ carrying out regular inspections to detect simple faults, such as frayed cables or cracked plugs

☐ reporting and clearly marking faulty equipment and taking it out of use until it is repaired.

This means that, as a therapist, you are responsible for the equipment you use.

EQUIPMENT CHECKLIST

- ☐ Check that it is safe.
- ☐ Keep equipment in good condition.
- ☐ Alert your salon to any equipment that needs attention.
- ☐ Keep careful records.
- ☐ Only use electrical equipment that you have been trained to use.

- ☐ Do not use any equipment you think might be unsafe.
- ☐ Use equipment according to instructions.
- ☐ Take all necessary safety precautions.

Your salon should provide all the necessary additional training in the use of their specific electrical equipment and in the safety procedures

Fuses

If an electrical appliance should fail, it is possible that it will fail in such a way as to draw a very heavy current from the mains supply. This current, converted to heat inside the equipment, may generate enough heat to cause a fire.

In order to prevent this happening, electrical appliances are fitted with fuses. A fuse consists of a small glass or ceramic tube with metal caps or contacts at each end.

Inside the body of the fuse, between the end caps, is connected a piece of wire. The wire is designed, through thickness, electrical resistance, etc to heat up enough to melt when the current flowing through it reaches a certain limit. In this way, if the appliance that the fuse is protecting fails and begins to draw too much current, the wire inside the fuse will heat up and melt, thereby cutting off the supply of power to the equipment. In a glass bodied fuse when this has happened you can see that the wire inside is now broken. A ceramic-bodied fuse may show discolouration due to the heat generated when the wire inside melts.

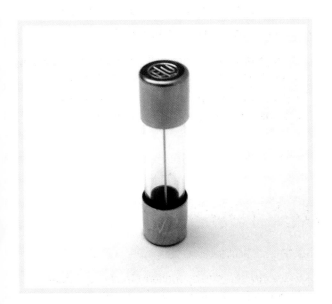

KEY POINT
The function of the fuse is to prevent an appliance drawing an excessively high current.

Choosing the right fuse rating

For the greatest degree of protection, we need the fuse to blow at a current loading just over the normal current drawn by a correctly-working appliance. As different appliances will have different power-ratings, and hence draw different amounts of current when working correctly, the correct fuse rating will also vary. To allow for this, fuses are available in a range of ratings.

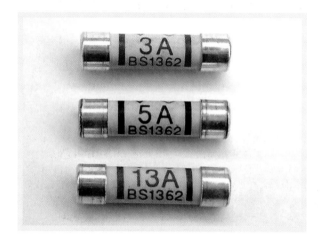

To decide what value of fuse to use, consult the appliance documentation, or look for information on the appliance itself. Do not assume that the fuse that has failed was of the correct rating – it may have been replaced with the wrong one by someone else.

If you know the power consumption of the appliance in watts, then you can calculate a suitable value for the fuse from the equation:

Current = Power/Voltage

As the mains voltage in the UK is 240 volts, a 700 watt appliance will draw 700/250 (or 2.8) amps of current. This is just less than a 3A fuse, and so a 3A fuse should be selected. Similarly we would use a:

- 5 amp fuse with an appliance between 750 and 1000 watts

- 13 amp fuse for appliances between 1000 and 3000 watts

If the fuse blows repeatedly:

- do not replace it with a higher value

- disconnect the equipment and get it checked by a suitably qualified electrician.

KEY POINT

Fuses come in 3A, 5A and 13A ratings. Use the right value – the fuse is there to protect you and your clients.

The correct wiring of a mains plug

In the UK new electrical products must, by law, come fitted with a mains plug. Most now come with a moulded plug which cannot be opened. A plug may need attention because it is damaged, or a fuse has blown. If you need to replace the fuse in a moulded plug, the fuse carrier can be levered out with a small screwdriver. A fuse of the same rating should be used to replace the blown fuse, and you should find out why the fuse blew. A damaged plug should be changed immediately as it is a safety risk. If the appliance is on premises to which members of the public have access then it should be PAT tested (Portable Appliance Testing) by a qualified electrician before use.

The colour-coding of the wires

If you were to unscrew the cover of the plug and remove it, the layout of the connections and wires inside would be like this.

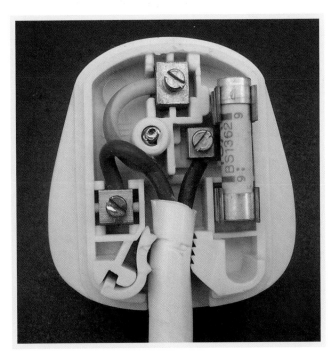

The fuse is on the right hand side. The three colours of wire used in the flex should be blue for neutral (N), brown for live (L), and green and yellow for earth (E). Some devices may only have the live and neutral wires, and no earth wire. These devices are called 'double-insulated' devices and they do not require an earth wire.

The terminal on the bottom right next to the fuse should be connected to the live (brown) cable. The left hand terminal should be connected to the neutral (blue) cable, and the top terminal should be connected to the earth (green and yellow) cable.

An easy way to remember the correct positions of the wires is:

BL – BLue – Bottom Left

BR – BRown – Bottom Right

At the bottom of the plug, where the cable enters, is either a small screw-down clamp, or a tight gap through which the cable fits. This is called the cable grip and its function is to prevent the wires inside becoming pulled out of their terminals if the cable is tugged on. The cable grip must hold the cable firmly in order for the plug to be safe.

Contraindications and sensitivity tests for electrical treatments

Before undertaking any treatment with a client, the therapist should always ensure the safety of the client and appropriateness of the treatment. See Chapter One for the contraindications that apply generally to all skin treatments. In addition, for electrical treatments, specific contraindications include:

- ☐ heart disease – a weak heart may not be able to cope with the increased blood flow stimulated by the electrical current
- ☐ hypersensitive skin – increased circulation may cause irritation and worsening of broken capillaries
- ☐ epilepsy – electrical treatment may cause an epileptic episode
- ☐ pregnancy – do not apply an electric current through the body
- ☐ diabetes – due to loss of skin sensation and bruising
- ☐ metal pins and plates
- ☐ loss of skin sensation (see below for tactile and thermal sensitivity tests)
- ☐ acute rheumatism
- ☐ osteoporosis
- ☐ trapped, pinched nerve.

In addition to consideration of general and treatment-specific contraindications, appropriate sensitivity tests should be performed. The purpose of sensitivity tests is to ensure that the client has normal, unimpaired sensitivity to stimuli, such as heat, pressure, etc, that provide warning against overexposure to the effects of some treatments. For electrical treatments, there are two important sensitivity tests that should be performed.

Nerve (tactile) sensitivity test

Before using an electrical treatment that stimulates the muscles, such as the faradic treatment, you must make sure that your client's sensory nerves are responding. Failure to do so could result in damaged facial muscles caused by the use of too high a current.

1. Ask your client to close their eyes.

2. Take a sharp object, such as an orange wood stick (rough), and then a soft object, such as cotton wool (smooth), and place them alternately on your client's skin.

3. Ask your client to say which is the rough and which is the smooth object.

– If your client can tell the difference, they have good sensitivity and you can proceed with the treatment.

– If your client cannot tell the difference, do not proceed; the treatment is then contraindicated.

Thermal sensitivity test

Before using an electrical heat treatment, such as infra red, you must make sure that your client's skin can differentiate between hot and cold sensations.

1. Fill two test tubes – one with hot water and one with cold water.

2. Place the test tubes alternately against your client's skin.

3. Ask your client to say which is the hot tube and which is the cold.

If your client can feel the sensation of heat, and can tell the difference between the tubes, then you can proceed with the treatment.

If your client cannot feel the difference, especially the feel of the hot tube, the treatment is contraindicated.

Electrical treatments and first aid

Because of the nature of electrical equipment which may, in an accident, cause either the therapist or the client to suffer electrical shock, burns or general shock,

it is essential that you understand the guide to basic first aid and emergency procedure contained in Chapter 1. A therapist cannot administer first aid unless they are qualified to do so. However, it is very useful to know what to do, and you may consider taking a first aid qualification.

First aid

A therapist should not give first aid unless qualified to do so, but should know the procedure for obtaining first aid.

ENDPOINTS
By the end of this topic, you should understand:

☐ the Health and Safety at Work Act 1974

☐ the Electricity at Work Act 1992

☐ fuses

☐ the correct wiring of a mains plug

☐ sensitivity tests for electrical treatments

☐ electrical treatments and first aid.

Topic 5: Galvanism: desincrustation and iontophoresis

Galvanism is an electrical treatment that passes a direct current through the skin. It can be used on all skin types, and its particular effects depend on the polarity used:

- A negatively charged active electrode with an active desincrustation gel product causes an alkaline reaction and deep cleansing effect (desincrustation).

- A positively charged active electrode with a positively charged gel or a negatively charged active electrode with a negatively charged gel, causes the active ingredients to be absorbed into the skin (iontophoresis).

Generally, desincrustation is a deep-cleanse, extracting treatment, while iontophoresis (or ionisation) passes substances into the skin to hydrate and nourish it. These treatments work on the principle that opposite poles attract, while like poles repel each other.

Effects of desincrustation

- Alkaline reaction (saponification).
- Opens the pores
- Softens the skin
- Dissolves sebum and deep cleanses
- Increases blood and lymph circulation

Effects of iontophoresis

- Acidic reaction on the skin
- Moisturises and hydrates by introducing active substances deeper into the skin than is normally possible without the use of galvanic current
- Firms and tightens the skin
- Decreases vascularity – taking blood supply away from the skin
- Refines large pores and closes pores after treatment

Desincrustation and iontophoresis are generally used as separate treatments but can be used in combination with each other, with desincrustation as the first treatment to deep cleanse the skin followed by iontophoresis to close the pores.

General effects of the galvanic current

The general benefits that a client is likely to notice after galvanic treatment are:

- stimulation through increased circulation
- improved skin colour

Safety precautions for galvanic treatments

- Check contraindications
- Check the machine is in good working order and has no loose wires or cracked plugs
- Check the machine is placed on a safe surface, e.g. a professional trolley
- Check there is no water on the trolley
- Prepare the skin appropriately, including tactile sensitivity test
- Check the machine on yourself first
- Talk to the client throughout the treatment
- Keep the electrodes moving throughout the treatment

Specific contraindications

In addition to general contraindications (see Chapter 1) and those for electrical treatments (see Topic 4 above), there are some specific contraindications to be aware of for galvanic treatments:

- sinusitis
- asthma
- loss of skin sensation (see Topic 4, tactile sensitivity test, which should be carried out before treatment)
- highly vascular or sensitive skin for desincrustation (however iontophoresis can help)
- braces, a large number of metal fillings or metal pins or plates in the face/head.

Preparing for galvanic treatments

1. Discuss the treatment beforehand with your client:

    – check for contraindications

    – explain the sequence of the treatment

    – describe to the client the sensations that they may experience, such as a metallic taste if they have metallic fillings (see Specific contraindications above), or a slight tingling in the skin. Ask your client to tell you if they experience these sensations. You can use this information together with careful visual observation to judge duration and intensity of treatment and the point at which to turn the current down. In the case of galvanism, providing the client can feel the 'prickle' of the current you can be assured that the machine is working and the current is flowing – therefore there is no reason to increase the intensity any further. This usually happens at a maximum of 1–2 amperes.

    – explain that if they feel uncomfortable, they should tell you and you will then reduce the amperage (intensity) or stop the treatment. The treatment should cause only gentle skin stimulation.

2. Test your client for skin sensitivity using the tactile sensitivity test (see page 262 above).

3. Ask your client to remove all jewellery and any other metal accessories worn, eg hair clips, and remove any of your own.

4. Check all the electrical equipment.

5. Make sure your client is lying down comfortably and the area of the skin to be treated is thoroughly cleansed and free of oil.

6. Apply the necessary gel or cream (see below).

The electrodes

The active or working electrode attached to the galvanic machine is the one you use to perform the treatment. There are several types of active electrodes:

☐   metal rollers

☐   metal ball electrodes – usually used for desincrustation

☐   tweezers or forceps

☐   rod with disc applicator heads

The passive or indifferent electrode, also attached to the galvanic machine, completes the circuit and is held by your client or placed on their body, generally behind their shoulder or strapped to their arm. This electrode is covered in a pre-dampened viscose sponge and should remain in contact with your client's body until the current is switched off.

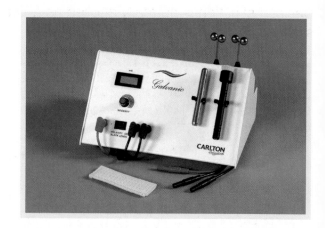

Using the electrodes

How you use the electrodes will depend upon the therapy you are giving

Desincrustation

☐ Move the active electrode over the face in small, smooth, circular movements.

☐ Apply with a firm, even pressure.

☐ Turn the current up slowly according to the amount of resistance in different parts of the face; for instance, lower the intensity of the current when working on the bony areas.

☐ Turn the current down slowly at the end of the treatment.

☐ Ensure that the electrodes are kept moving and remain in contact with the client's skin until the current has been zeroed.

Iontophoresis

☐ Move the active rollers over the face in long even stokes ensuring they do not touch each other

☐ Apply with a firm, even pressure.

☐ Turn the current up slowly according to the amount of resistance in different parts of the face; for instance, lower the intensity of the current when working on the bony areas.

☐ Turn the current down slowly at the end of the treatment.

☐ Ensure that the electrodes are kept moving and remain in contact with the client's skin until the current has been zeroed.

The desincrustation treatment

Desincrustination is normally applied as a deep-cleansing treatment, such as after a facial steam.

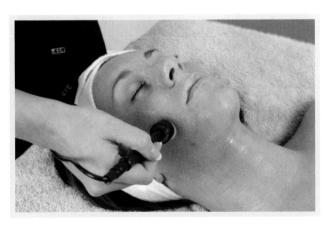

1. Moisten the skin well and lightly apply a negatively charged desincrustation gel onto the skin. Always follow the manufacturer's instructions.

2. Apply the electrode to the skin of the cheek and switch the machine on, increasing the intensity slowly. Allow about 30 seconds for the resistance of oily, congested skin to be overcome.

3. Use the electrodes as described above. This treatment should work well even on very low

amperage, up to 0.6 milliamps (mA). As the galvanic current works by a process of attraction to its opposite pole, working from positive to negative, there is no need to use high intensity.

4. Timing should be about 3 to 10 minutes depending upon the condition of the skin.

5. Ensure that the skin remains moist to allow the galvanic current to work and avoid skin irritation.

6. Conclude the treatment by slowly reducing the intensity to zero, removing the electrodes and switching the machine off.

7. After treatment, wipe off any remaining desincrustation gel with cotton wool or sponges, until the skin looks clean and gently stimulated and all traces of product are removed.

8. Follow with any further treatments, such as manual extraction or removal of comedones by vacuum suction.

9. Clean the electrodes with sanitising fluid immediately after use.

The iontophoresis (ionisation) treatment

If iontophoresis is being incorporated in a full facial treatment it should be performed last.

1. Apply a positively charged substance to the skin, always following the manufacturer's instructions.

Safety

Most galvanic substances are positively charged for iontophoresis and negatively charged for desincrustation. However sometimes manufacturer's reverse the polarity. It is vital, therefore, when performing galvanism that you always check the labelling of the product and follow the manufacturer's instructions.

2. Using the same pole as the charged substance, use the electrodes as described in 'Using the electrodes' above to repel the active substance into the body tissues towards the opposite pole, which is placed behind the client's shoulder blade or in their hand.

3. Treatment time is approximately 3–10 minutes. High intensity is not needed. Sensitive skin will require less time or lower intensity to avoid irritation.

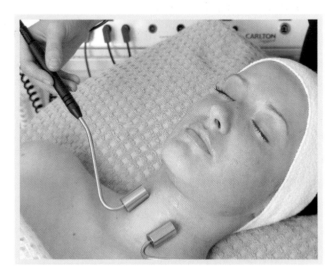

4. Conclude the treatment by reducing the intensity to zero, removing the electrode(s) and turning the equipment off. Sanitise the electrodes immediately.

5. Blot the skin if necessary and advise the client not to apply make-up for 12–24 hours afterwards.

Safety

Never allow the skin to become dry, as this could result in a galvanic burn. Never hold the electrodes in one place always keep them moving for the same reason.

Concluding the galvanic treatment

1. Detach all electrodes and sanitise and store them appropriately.

2. Do not apply make-up for a minimum of 12–24 hours, to allow the skin to gain maximum benefit from the treatment.

3. Be sure to update client records after electrical treatments.

4. Give the client suitable skin and home care advice.

ENDPOINTS

By the end of this topic, you should understand:

☐ the effects of desincrustination and iontophoresis

☐ safety precautions for galvanic treatments

☐ how to prepare for and perform galvanic treatments.

Topic 6: High-frequency treatments

High-frequency machines use an oscillating alternating current whose frequency is high enough to warm the tissues. It can also produce ozone which destroys the surface bacteria that can cause pustules and acne, producing a drying and healing effect on the skin. High-frequency treatments can be either direct or indirect.

- direct – the high-frequency current passes directly into the client's skin through an electrode

or

- indirect – the high-frequency current discharges from the client to the therapist's hands at the point of contact during a gentle massage.

Direct

Direct treatments are most beneficial for oily, blemished, pustular, sallow or sluggish skins. They are used to:

- produce ozone to destroy bacteria, dry the skin and help to heal pustules
- increase circulation
- encourage desquamation
- improve skin colour
- stimulate cell renewal
- stimulate subcutaneous tissue and blood circulation to bring fresh nutrients to the surface and eliminate waste
- stimulate sensory nerve endings.

Indirect

Indirect treatments are most beneficial for dry, mature skins as they work by gently moisturising the skin through a soothing massage. They are used to:

- relax and relieve tension through localised warmth
- stimulate subcutaneous tissue and blood circulation to bring fresh nutrients to the surface and eliminate waste
- stimulate sensory nerve endings
- improve skin texture and colour through desquamation
- improve skin texture and moisture levels through absorption of nourishing creams.

Contraindications specific to high-frequency treatments

In addition to the contraindications given in Chapter 1 and those for electrical treatments given above in Topic 4, specific contraindications for high-frequency treatments are:

- susceptibility to headaches and migraines
- high blood pressure or treatment for defective circulation, e.g. oedema
- pacemaker
- highly strung, nervous disposition
- asthma
- sinus blockage
- skin infection
- excessive number of metallic fillings
- loss of skin sensation (see Topic 4, tactile sensitivity test, which should be carried out before treatment).

Safety precautions for high frequency treatments

- Check contraindications
- Remove any jewellery and metal accessories, e.g. hair clips from both you and your client
- Check the machine is in good working order and has no loose wires or cracked plugs, etc
- Check the machine is placed on a safe surface such as a professional trolley
- Check there is no water on the trolley
- Prepare the skin appropriately
- Explain the treatment to the client
- Check the machine on yourself first
- Talk to the client throughout the treatment
- Ensure the electrode is in contact with the skin prior to switching the machine on
- During treatment, make sure that neither you nor your client is in contact with any metal, such as a trolley, stool or couch
- Do not touch your client, their clothing, covering, the gauze or the couch during treatment
- Keep the electrodes moving throughout the treatment and in full contact with the skin unless sparking is required
- Turn the frequency down on bony areas
- Ensure that the frequency is at zero and the machine turned off before removing the electrode from the client's skin
- Ensure the electrodes are sanitised and placed in a sanitising cabinet after treatment.

Preparing for high-frequency treatments

1. Discuss the treatment with your client first, and explain the treatment sequence to them, including the use of the current, and the noise of the machine, such as the loud buzzing that occurs with high-frequency treatment which can be disturbing to some clients, the smell of ozone, and the nature of sparking (see 'Safety'). Do not begin the treatment until your client understands and is relaxed about what will happen.

2. Ask your client to remove all jewellery and remove any jewellery you may be wearing yourself.

3. Complete all the electrical checks on the equipment and check that the intensity dial is set at zero and the machine is switched off.

4. Make sure your client's skin is thoroughly cleansed before treatment.

5. Make sure that your client is lying in a comfortable position before starting.

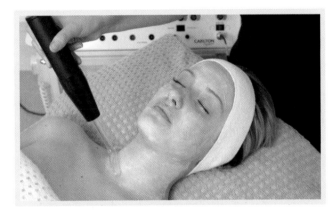

The electrodes

Different glass electrodes are inserted into an ebonite handle that is attached to the machine by a cord. The most commonly used electrode for direct treatments is:

☐ the mushroom surface electrode – in different sizes to suit different parts of the face and neck.

Other electrodes used in direct treatments are:

☐ the roller – for larger areas, such as the back

☐ the horseshoe or T-shaped electrode – for the back of the neck and shoulders

☐ the fulgurator – to spark pustules

☐ the rake – for the scalp and hair.

In indirect treatments the electrode the client holds is:

☐ the saturator electrode – a glass and metal rod attached to the machine to complete the circuit.

Using the electrodes for H-F direct treatment

1. Apply powder to give 'slip' to the surface of the skin

2. Turn the machine on only when the electrode is already touching your client's skin.

3. Use small circular movements, starting on the neck area, or on the forehead using the small mushroom electrode.

4. Do not press hard, glide the electrode lightly – the lighter the contact, the more stimulating the treatment.

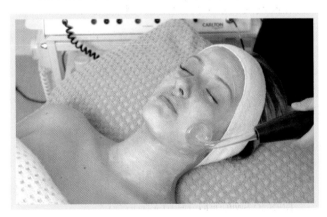

5. Do not use the electrode at an angle. Take special care around the nose to keep the plane of the electrode flat. It may be preferable to switch to a smaller electrode.

6. Check with your client to ensure that the treatment is tolerable at all times. If your client has an adverse reaction, turn down and then zero the current before removing the electrode.

7. Lower the intensity of the current over bony areas.

8. Ensure that the electrode remains in contact with the skin at all times until the end of the treatment and until after the intensity has been zeroed.

9. Remove the powder with damp cotton wool and tone.

10. The treatment should not exceed 10 minutes.

Safety

When 'sparking' the pustules, or scar tissue or to activate a sluggish, sallow complexion using the fulgurator, slightly lift the electrode from the skin (never more that 6mm) for a very short time and lift on and off up to 4 times only, very quickly. The current intensifies as it jumps across the gap between the electrode and skin so should be used with caution, otherwise it may be destructive to the tissues.

High-frequency (HF) indirect treatment

1. Apply cream or oil sufficient to last for the whole massage and according to the client's skin type over the face, neck and chest.

2. Give your client the indifferent, saturator electrode to hold throughout the treatment.

3. Place one hand on your client's cheek before turning on the machine with the other hand and raising the current to an acceptable frequency, i.e. they should be able to feel the slight prickle of the current through your finger tips.

4. With both hands, perform the facial massage routine using all the classical massage movements except tapotement. Superficial movements give a stimulating reaction, while deep movements are more relaxing. Treat the bony, sensitive areas, such as the forehead, lightly to avoid discomfort. Take care when using a lesser part of the hand as the current intensifies in those areas of the hand which remain in contact with the client.

5. At least one hand must be in contact with your client's skin at all times until the end of the treatment and after the intensity has been zeroed.

6. Do not work too near your client's eyes or mouth.

7. Check with your client that the treatment is comfortable at all times. If they have an adverse reaction, turn down the intensity and zero the current before removing your other hand.

8. At the end of the massage, remove one hand to turn down the current and switch off the machine. Then you can remove your other hand.

9. Time taken should not exceed a normal 20-minute facial massage.

After high-frequency treatments

1. Wipe your client's skin clean with damp cotton wool or sponges to remove any remaining product.

2. Remove, clean and sterilise the electrodes used. Clean and wipe over the machine and ebony handle with sanitiser.

3. Keep the skin clean and do not apply make-up for as long as possible after the treatment in order to allow the skin time to gain maximum benefit from it.

4. Be sure to update client records after electrical treatments.

5. Give the client suitable skin and homecare advice.

ENDPOINTS

By the end of this topic, you should understand:

☐ the uses of direct and indirect high-frequency treatments

☐ contraindications to high-frequency treatments

☐ how to prepare for high-frequency treatments

☐ how to perform high-frequency treatments.

Topic 7: Faradic treatments

Faradism is known as a passive exercise treatment, as it exercises the muscles by passing an electrical current through them without conscious effort by the client. The current causes the muscle to contract in the 'stimulating' period and relax in the stimulation interval to prevent muscle fatigue.

Faradism is especially beneficial to ageing or sagging skins with dropped contours and as a preventative measure to promote a healthy and toned skin appearance. It improves the general contours of the face.

The effects of faradic treatments

Faradism is used to:

- [ ] improve muscle tone, by tightening and firming sagging muscles, enhancing and defining existing features

- [ ] increases local blood circulation and metabolism, bringing nourishment to the skin

- [ ] refine fine lines by improving facial contours

- [ ] stimulate nerve endings

- [ ] re-educate muscles that have been inactive

- [ ] increase blood and lymph flow, removing toxins and waste

- [ ] increase the energy-producing chemical ATP.

Contraindications specific to facial faradic treatments

In addition to the contraindications given in Chapter 1 and those for electrical treatments given above in Topic 4, specific contraindications for facial faradism treatment are:

- [ ] loss of skin sensation (see Topic 4, tactile sensitivity test, which should be performed before treatment)

- [ ] muscular disorders

- [ ] highly nervous clients

- [ ] metal pins and plates

- [ ] excessive fillings

- [ ] high blood pressure

- [ ] Bell's palsy

- [ ] Neuralgia and any dysfunction of the nervous system

- [ ] migraine sufferers

- [ ] sinus congestion

- [ ] any area of the face where severe discomfort is experienced during treatment

- [ ] sunburn

- [ ] pacemakers

- [ ] circulatory disorders

- [ ] botox

- [ ] dermal fillers.

Note: The stimulation of the nerve endings will produce a sensation of tingling, which you should warn your clients about prior to increasing the current to achieve a contraction.

Electrodes used for faradic treatments

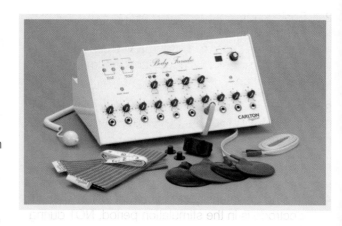

There are several different types of electrode that can be used for faradic treatment:

☐ an indifferent or passive electrode, dampened with saline solution and attached to the client, with an active disc electrode covered in lint or heavy gauze soaked in saline solution to increase conductivity

☐ a twin electrode containing both a passive and active electrode, moistened with a saline solution.

Preparing for faradic treatment

1. Discuss all aspects of the treatment with your client, including the tingling sensation mentioned above.

2. Carry out a tactile sensitivity test.

3. Check all the electrical equipment you will be using.

4. Make sure your client is lying comfortably in a fairly upright position so that the muscles adopt a natural position with gravity.

5. Thoroughly cleanse your client's skin and ensure all cream and/or oil is removed from the skin's surface before commencing the treatment. This treatment is usually included as part of a full facial treatment.

6. Make sure you are in a position to see and adjust the controls easily.

Carrying out faradic treatment

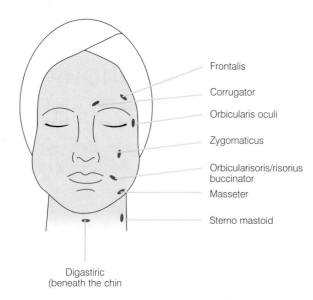

Frontalis

Corrugator

Orbicularis oculi

Zygomaticus

Orbicularisoris/risorius buccinator

Masseter

Sterno mastoid

Digastiric
(beneath the chin

Safety

Always follow the manufacturer's instructions for the machine you are using for any faradic treatment, as these can vary considerably.

1. Turn on the machine then position the form of electrode you are using before turning up the frequency dial.

2. Soak cotton wool in saline solution (1% dilution of salt in water) then place over the electrode before placing on the skin. This improves conductivity and muscle point response and reduces skin irritation.

3. Position the electrode carefully on the muscle motor points (see illustration on opposite page) starting with the neck. The more accurately the electrode is placed, the stronger the contraction and the smaller the amount of irritation.

4. Turn up the intensity of the current ONLY when the electrode is in the stimulation period, NOT during the interval.

5. Increase the intensity until a contraction is seen. A full contraction should be seen in the muscle and it is vital that the electrode is held firmly against the muscle as it contracts. Repeat 6–8 times per muscle.

6. Do not work too near the mouth if the client has a large number of metal fillings or is wearing braces on their teeth. Treatment is most effective and comfortable around the outer borders of the face. If treatment is specifically required in the lip area, regulate the intensity carefully to avoid discomfort. Most treatment will be on the antigravity muscles, i.e. those that show the first signs of ageing.

7. Progress up to the mandible, cheek and eye areas, applying eight contractions on each motor point. For general firming, follow the sequence:

    – sternomastoid

    – platysma

    – masseter

    – zygomatic

    – risorius

    – orbicularis oris

    – levators of the lip

    – eye area

    – orbicularis oculi

    – corrugator

    – frontalis

8. Turn the current down before moving the electrode.

9. Alter the treatment according to careful observation and client feedback and gradually increase the number of contractions per muscle to a maximum of eight.

10. Keep the electrode in contact with your client's skin until the intensity has been zeroed.

After faradic treatment

1. Remove any remaining saline with damp cotton wool.

2. Wipe the electrode with sanitiser and place it in a sanitising cabinet.

3. Continue with any further treatment.

4. Be sure to update client records after electrical treatments.

ENDPOINTS
By the end of this topic, you should understand:

☐ the effects of faradic treatments

☐ contraindications to faradic treatments

☐ how to prepare for a faradic treatment

☐ how to carry out a faradic treatment.

Topic 8: Microcurrent treatments

Originating as a sports physiotherapy and Bell's palsy treatment, Microcurrent Electrical Neurotransmuscular Stimulation (MENS) has been successfully adapted to use its toning and firming effect as a cosmetic treatment to rejuvenate and recontour facial muscles. It works by using a very low frequency microcurrent to stimulate the golgi tendon organ, which helps protect muscles and keeps them toned and active. Microcurrent treatment is gentle and relaxing and suitable for all ages and skins. Treatment time is up to one hour, with a routine of several treatments a week for several weeks recommended, then moving to a less frequent maintenance programme.

Effects of microcurrent treatments

Microcurrent treatments are used to:

☐ improve muscle tone by tightening and firming sagging muscles, refining fine lines, enhancing and defining existing features

☐ increase blood and lymph circulation and metabolism, removing toxins and waste and bringing nourishment to the skin

☐ stimulate exhausted skin, improving colour

☐ increase cellular regeneration, delaying signs of ageing.

Contraindications specific to microcurrent treatments

In addition to the contraindications given in Chapter 1 and those for electrical treatments given in Topic 4 above, specific contraindications for microcurrent treatment are:

☐ loss of skin sensation (see Topic 4, tactile sensitivity test, which should be performed before treatment)

☐ muscular disorders, such as muscular sclerosis

☐ metal pins and plates

☐ excessive dental fillings

☐ pacemakers

☐ heart conditions

☐ diabetes

☐ varicose veins

☐ Neuralgia, migraines or any dysfunction of the nervous system

☐ dermal fillers or collagen treatments

☐ recent Botox injections

☐ pustular acne

☐ facial implants

☐ when muscle relaxants have been prescribed.

Preparing for microcurrent treatments

1. Check the client's record card.

2. Discuss all aspects of the treatment with your client, including the tingling sensation that may result.

2. Sanitise your hands.

3. Carry out a tactile sensitivity test.

4. Check all the electrical equipment you will be using.

5. Test the machine on yourself.

6. Make sure your client is lying comfortably in a fairly upright position so that the muscles adopt a natural position with gravity.

7. Ask the client to remove all jewellery and take off any of your own.

8. Thoroughly cleanse and warm your client's skin to relax the tissues and aid conductivity, and ensure all cream and/or oil is removed from the skin's surface before commencing the treatment. This treatment is often included as part of a full facial treatment.

9. Make sure you are in a position to see and adjust the controls easily.

Electrodes used for microcurrent treatments

There are several different types of electrodes that can be used for microcurrent treatment. They may be either microcurrent electrode pads, probes (single or dual), gloves, hands (as in indirect high frequency treatment), or a combination.

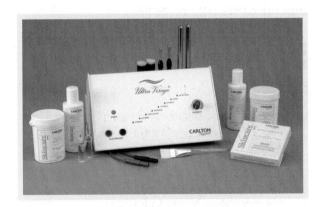

Carrying out microcurrent treatments

Safety

Always follow the instructions appropriate to the machine you are using for any microcurrent treatment, as these may vary considerably.

1. Apply an electrolytic gel to the client's skin to improve conductivity and reduce skin irritation.

2. Select the waveform, frequency and current according to the client's skin condition. Unlike faradic treatments, microcurrent causes little or no visible contraction of the facial muscles, and so, for their comfort, you must be sensitive to the client's responses to the current.

3. Use single probes or pads to stimulate specific muscles and produce a lifting effect. On larger muscles such as those along the jaw area use dual probes, moving the larger toward the smaller in a smooth, even motion.

After microcurrent treatments

1. Remove any remaining gel or saline with damp cotton wool.

2. Wipe the electrodes with a sanitiser and place in a sanitising cabinet.

3. Continue with any further treatment, such as ionisation

4. Remember to provide appropriate after-care advice – in general clients should avoid the application of facial creams or make-up for an hour after treatment.

5. Be sure to update client records after electrical treatments.

ENDPOINTS

By the end of this topic, you should understand:

☐ the effects of microcurrent treatments

☐ contraindications to microcurrent treatments

☐ how to prepare for a microcurrent treatment

☐ how to carry out a microcurrent treatment.

Topic 9: Vacuum suction

Vacuum suction is used to stimulate lymphatic drainage and the vacuum massage movements also increase vascular circulation. It is beneficial to all skin types, especially:

- oily, blemished skin
- dry, dehydrated skin
- mature skin.

The method of vacuum suction can be adapted for the different skin types. Mature skin generally benefits from an intermittent pulse action.

Vacuum suction is usually applied after cleansing as a deep-cleansing treatment, or used to intensely massage the skin. The first treatment should be carried out with careful checking of the skin's reaction. If successful the treatment can be repeated, preferably about three times a week in a ten-treatment course, increasing the length of treatment time to a maximum of 10 minutes for mature skins and 15 minutes for all other skin types.

General effects of vacuum suction

Vacuum suction treatment is used to:

- improve elimination and absorption of waste products through the lymphatic system
- deep cleanse by removing skin blockages and congestion – sometimes used in conjunction with ozone steaming and galvanic desincrustation
- improve skin texture through desquamation
- nourish skin and improve skin colour by stimulating circulation
- maintain skin firmness and ease out fine lines
- hydrate and moisturise.

Contraindications specific to vacuum suction treatment

In addition to the contraindications given in Chapter 1 and those for electrical treatments given above in Topic 4, specific contraindications for vacuum suction treatment are:

- broken capillaries
- fine, sensitive
- loose, crepey skin
- acne rosecea and vulgaris
- delicate skin around the eyes
- bruised or broken skin
- bony areas
- loss of skin sensation (see Topic 4, tactile sensitivity test, which should be performed before treatment).

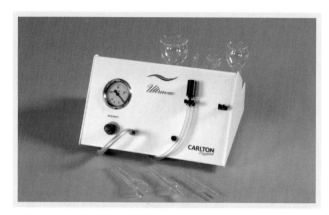

The applicator/ ventouse

The applicator/ventouse is a perspex/glass cup, attached to an electrically driven vacuum pump, which creates a partial vacuum when placed on the skin. Ventouse come in varying shapes and sizes to suit different parts of the face or different functions. Ventouse with:

☐ large openings, 10cm or above, use low levels of vacuum to treat the upper chest and back, and areas of subcutaneous tissues

☐ 5cm openings are suitable for neck and firm skin on very low levels of vacuum

☐ flattened narrow openings are suitable for lines and flexure folds for temporary easing of lines

☐ the smallest openings are used for comedone extractions, fine lines and sensitive skin (higher levels of vacuum).

Some applicators have a small hole in the side of the ventouse that you can cover with your finger to create the vacuum, then uncover to release the vacuum and break the seal with the skin.

The amount of negative pressure used to create the vacuum is varied to suit the condition and flaccidity of the skin. There should be no more than 20% lift in the tissues as bruising or capillary damage could occur.

Preparing for vacuum suction treatment

1. Discuss all aspects of the treatment with your client.

2. Check all electrical equipment first, including the ventouse for cracks or chips on the rim.

3. Make sure your client's skin is cleansed, then apply oil or cream as an appropriate lubricant for the skin type.

4. Test the vacuum pressure on your own skin first and adjust if necessary.

5. Carry out the treatment.

The gliding method

1. Place the ventouse on the skin of the decolleté and turn on the machine.

2. Slightly lift and use gliding strokes towards the lymph nodes.

3. Break the suction of the ventouse by placing your finger under the rim of the ventouse and gently depressing the skin, or releasing your finger over the hole in the ventouse.

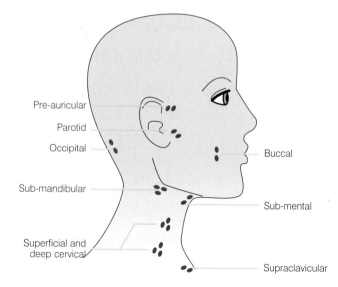

Safety

Never pull the ventouse directly off the skin. Always ensure that the suction has been broken first by taking the finger off the hole on the side of the ventouse to release the vacuum.

4. Overlap the strokes by half a width of the ventouse to ensure that the whole area is covered. Each strip of tissue should be treated 3–6 times prior to moving on by the width of half a ventouse.

5. Follow the pattern of strokes indicated in the diagram, working towards the lymph nodes.

6. Observe your client's skin reaction, checking that your client remains comfortable throughout the treatment.

7. After the general treatment, use the specialised applicators on the central panel to remove comedones where necessary or on fine lines to plump up the tissue.

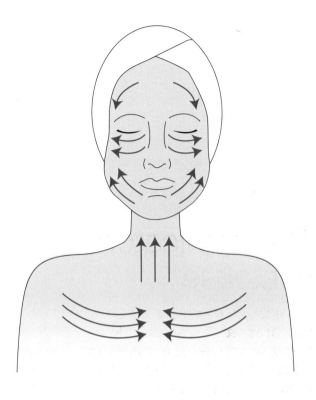

The pulsating method (tapping)

Tapping is particularly beneficial when used over the lines of the forehead, especially with the flat applicator.

1. A pulsating or tapping effect can be obtained by using either a ventouse with an air hole, and rapidly lifting and replacing your finger over the hole or a pulsed air machine using two applicators in unison to stimulate the skin gently.

2. The effect can be produced with the ventouse static or during gliding movements. If the ventouse is static, do not concentrate for too long on one area as this can cause bruising and blood spots on the skin.

3. When using a comedone extractor applicator, place it over the comedone and lift rapidly on and off the area until the comedone has eased or been extracted. Some ventouse have a hole, in which case the tapping procedure can be used.

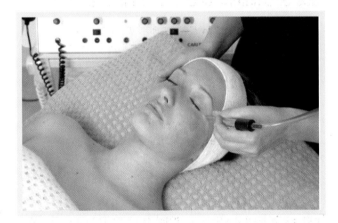

4. Position the client to start treatment on the decollette:

    – Use the vacuum in the gliding method working inward toward the lymphatic and thoracic ducts on the chest

    – Move up and treat the platysma muscle area using diagonal strokes to the base of the throat, avoiding pressure on the windpipe (trachea) draining lymph to the deep and superficial cervical and submandiblar nodes in the neck.

    – working with both hands in unison or alternately, work up from the mandible to behind the ear towards the anterior and posterior auricular nodes

    – continue with treating the face, adapting the ventouses to your client's features and skin condition, ending by draining outwards on the forehead towards the anterior auricular lymph nodes.

    – Change to a smaller ventouse to treat any other areas required, such as the chin, upper lip and laughter lines, or to treat blocked pores.

5. Treatment is applied towards the lymph nodes to encourage lymphatic drainage.

After vacuum suction treatment

1. Use damp cotton wool or sponges to remove any remaining product from your client's skin.

2. Continue with any further treatment if vacuum suction is part of a larger treatment.

3. Detach, clean and thoroughly cleanse all tubing in detergent and place it in a sanitised container. Detach and clean the ventouse in detergent first .then place in a sanitising cabinet.

4. Be sure to update client records, as after any electrical treatment.

ENDPOINTS

By the end of this topic, you should understand:

☐   the general effects of vacuum treatments

☐   contraindications to vacuum treatment

☐   how to prepare for vacuum treatments

☐   how to perform vacuum treatments.

Topic 10:
Infra-red treatments

Infra-red rays work by penetrating the superficial epidermis, producing heat, warming and soothing the body tissues. In addition to their therapeutic effects on the skin, infra-red treatments generally help people to relax and give them a feeling of well-being.

Infra-red may also be used in conjunction with a hot-oil mask (see Chapter 3) which is particularly suitable for dry and dehydrated skin as the oil is absorbed directly and quickly into the skin during treatment, improving elasticity and texture. It is also suitable for crepey, finely lined, mature skin. The heat lamp is especially beneficial for clients with aching muscles and areas of tension. Infra-red treatment is also often used as a preparatory treatment before massage.

General effects of infra-red treatments

Infra-red treatments are used to:

- increase circulation, thereby nourishing the skin and improving waste removal including increased activity of sweat glands

- heat the blood and warm the tissues, creating erythema

- dilate the pores

- relax tense muscles

- preheat tissues prior to further treatment

- increase absorption of products

Contraindications specific to infra-red treatments

In addition to the contraindications given in Chapter 1 and those for electrical treatments given above in Topic 4, specific contraindications for infra-red treatments are:

- loss of skin sensation (see Topic 4, thermal sensitivity test, which should be carried out before treatment)

- areas of dilated capillaries (these must be covered with damp cotton wool pads to prevent heat penetration)

- hypersensitive skin

- diabetes

- sunburn

Safety precautions specific to heat-lamp treatment

Using a heat lamp creates more potential hazards in the salon.
Following a checklist can help ensure that your client enjoys the treatment safely.

CHECKLIST

1. Check the lamp, ensuring that:

   – there are no trailing, loose or frayed wires

   – there are no dents in the canopy of the lamp – this would cause the tissues to be heated unevenly creating 'hot spots'

   – the lamp has been warmed up away from the client (the lamp should be switched on at least 10-15 minutes before it is needed to reach its maximum intensity)

   – the lamp is positioned over the tripod leg and not directly above the client

   – the lamp has been tightened to prevent any movement once it is in position

   – the lamp should be placed a minimum of 50 cm away from the most prominent point on the area to be treated (and usually not further than 1m). For a reminder of the inverse square law, see opposite

   – you are following the manufacturer's instruction about use, distance and angle of the lamp

   – the lamp is clean, dust free and in good working order

   – the lamp is positioned safely away from the client in order to cool down.

2. Check that:

   – your client has removed contact lenses and all jewellery before treatment

   – your client's skin is suitable for infra-red treatment (see thermal sensitivity test and contraindications on page 262)

3. Protect your client's eyes with damp cotton wool pads that will absorb the rays.

4. Check your client's skin reaction throughout treatment.

5. Never leave your client alone during treatment.

6. Do not use the lamp for longer than the specified time.

Using hot-oil mask with infra-red lamp treatment

When using a hot-oil mask, soak the gauze with warm oil, such as almond oil, and place over the face before applying the lamp treatment.

Check that prominent areas, such as the nose tip, are covered, while allowing holes for the nostrils, and cover the eyes with eye pads. In all other respects follow the safety precautions in the checklist on the previous page. Leave the lamp for approximately 10 minutes (always follow the manufacturer's instructions) and stay with your client throughout the treatment. Only remove the mask after switching off and removing the lamp. Massage excess oil into the skin using the facial massage routine. Then remove any remaining oil with damp cotton wool, and apply a toner.

See Chapter 3, Topic 11 for details about hot-oil mask treatments and contraindications to them.

Safety and the inverse square law

The intensity of rays varies inversely with the square of the distance from the lamp. Thus, the intensity of radiation at 30cm is 4 times that at 60cm and 11 times that at 1m, so 1 minute at 30cm distance is the equivalent of 4 minutes at 60cm and 11 minutes at 1m.

Because of this you must always adhere to manufacturer's instructions on exposure time and distance of the lamp from the client's skin.

ENDPOINTS
By the end of this topic, you should understand:

☐ the general effects of infra-red treatment

☐ contraindications to infra-red treatment

☐ safety precautions for infra-red treatment

☐ the implications of the inverse square law for safe infra-red treatment.

Topic 11: Microdermabrasion

Microdermabrasion is an exfoliation treatment that uses a compressor and a low-pressure suction pump to deliver a controlled stream of micronised aluminium oxide crystals to the skin. Developed initially by dermatologists, it can now be used by beauty therapists to treat many different skin types, from thick, coarse skin to thin, ageing skin, for conditions ranging from reducing the signs of ageing to treating sun-damage and pigmentation disorders.

The levels of treatment

Microdermabrasion can be used at different levels to produce different effects according to the client's skin type:

- **Level 1** – exfoliates and helps remove comedones and milia
- **Level 2** – helps in the treatment of fine lines and wrinkles, pigmentation and acne scars, and complements the use of microcurrent treatment
- **Level 3** – helps in the treatment of scars, lip and frown lines and stretch marks.

The level of treatment must be selected by the therapist appropriately for the client's skin type and conditions.

How microdermabrasion works

The microdermabrasion machine consists of a compressor connected to a treatment probe, a container of fresh, sterile microcrystals and a container to collect waste crystals and exfoliated skin.

When the probe is pressed onto the client's skin a vacuum is created which draws fresh crystals from the container and down the tubes onto the skin, where they gently exfoliate the cells on the surface of the skin, before being sucked into the waste container.

General effects of microdermabrasion

Microdermabrasion is used to:

- Improve the skin's texture
- reduce fine lines and wrinkles
- refine acne-scarred skin or stretch marks
- remove skin congestion
- treat pigmentation disorders and age spots
- improve sun-damaged skin
- improve skin colour
- improve absorption rate of moisturising and other active ingredients.

Contraindications specific to microdermabrasion

In addition to the contraindications given in Chapter 1 and those for electrical treatments given above in Topic 4, specific contraindications for microdermabrasion treatments are:

- recent exfoliation treatments, such as chemical peels
- hepatitis, HIV or other disorders transmitted by body fluids
- haemophilia or the use of anti-coagulant medication
- diabetes
- asthma
- spastic conditions
- recent cosmetic or other surgery
- injections for personal enhancement
- hypersensitive skin
- haematoma
- moles, birthmarks, or keloid scarring
- loss of skin sensation (a tactile sensitivity test should be performed before treatment).

Preparing for the treatment

Perform a normal client assessment, taking account of the contraindications listed above, and communicating to the client the procedures, effects and possible after-effects of the proposed treatment. Microdermabrasion equipment can be noisy, and it is important to warn, and reassure, the client about this in advance. Then:

- check electrical safety of the machine.
- ensure that the waste crystal container is empty and any filters are clear
- fill the crystal container on the machine with fresh, dry crystals to the right level according to the manufacturer's instructions.
- reseal the container of fresh crystals to prevent them absorbing moisture or becoming contaminated.
- fit a new disposable (or sterile if reusable) applicator to the machine probe.
- test machine to ensure it is functioning correctly.
- sanitise your hands

Preparing your client

Having prepared for the treatment, you should next prepare your client by:

- ensuring that they are comfortable on the treatment couch and their clothing is covered with a clean towel
- asking them to remove any earrings or other facial jewellery
- cleansing, toning and drying their skin as the crystals will not work properly if they get damp)
- apply protective eyeshields to their eyes
- testing the suction setting of the machine on yourself.

Performing the treatment

Ensure that you are familiar with the manufacturer's guidelines for use of the machine and:

- turn on the machine
- adjust the suction setting on the compressor appropriately to the client's skin type, sensitivity and condition

- place the probe on their skin to begin the flow of crystals
- move the probe continuously across the skin
- follow the lines of lymphatic flow – on the face this should normally be from the centre outwards
- use the appropriate number of coatings for the client's skin type and sensitivity
- treat blemishes such as scarring or pigmentation marks individually.
- allow 50 to 60 minutes for a facial treatment
- after treatment, remove any remaining excess crystals
- apply a calming treatment mask to the skin.

After the treatment

After you have completed the treatment, you should:

- empty the used crystal container and dispose of used crystals appropriately, so as to ensure no cross-contamination with clean crystals
- check and clean/replace filters in the machine according to the manufacturer's recommendations
- dispose of used treatment heads or sanitise re-usable treatment heads appropriately
- update the client's record card
- provide your client with appropriate after-care advice.

After-care advice for clients

After completion of the treatment you should advise the client to:

- avoid exposure to the sun
- avoid tanning treatments
- use a daily application of a sunscreen of at least SPF30
- avoid all exfoliation treatments during the course of microdermabrasion treatments.

ENDPOINTS

By the end of this topic, you should understand:

- the benefits of microdermabrasion
- contraindications to microdermabrasion
- how to prepare for a microdermabrasion treatment
- how to perform a microdermabrasion treatment
- post treatment procedures
- aftercare advice for microdermabrasion treatments.

Characteristics of electrical treatments

Skin types and length of treatment (in minutes)

Treatment	Action/effects	Indications for use					
		Dry	Oily	Combination	Dehydrated	Mature	Sensitive
Galvanic desincrustation	Deep skin cleansing. Unblocks pores. Normalises skin's oil/water balance improves skin colour/texture/function.		3–10	3–10			
Galvanic iontophoresis/ionisation	Hydrates/moisturises Normalises skin balance Regenerates, soothes, calms. Improves skin's elasticity.	3–10	3–6	3–6	3–6	3–10	3
High-frequency direct method	Stimulates Germicidal		5–10	5–10			
High-frequency indirect method	Relaxation. Improves circulation.Nourishing	20			20	20	5–10
Faradism	Muscle stimulation and strengthening. Increases circulation. Refines lines	Each muscle to be contracted approx 6–8 times each					
Microcurrent	Improves cell regeneration/lymphatic flow. Re-educates inactive muscles. Boosts production of ATP	Full treatment approx 1 hour					
Vacuum suction	Cleanses/desquamates. Stimulates. Improves lymphatic circulation/drainage.	10–15	10–15	10–15	10–15	5–10	
Infra-red Hot oil masks	Prepares for massage Increases circulation. Dilates pores Relaxes muscles.Increases absorption.Relieves pain.	10			10	10	
Microdermabrasion	Exfoliates. Helps remove comedones/milia.Treats fine lines/wrinkles/pigmentation/scars. Prepares for higher treatments.	40–60	40–60	40–60	40–60	40–60	
Steaming. Normal or with herbs/essential oils	Relaxes. Softens/hydrates/cleanses/desquamates skin. Stimulates.	5	10	10	5	5	
Steaming with ozone	Dries. Heals. Anti-bacterial. Stimulates.		5–10	5–8			
Brush cleaning	Stimulating. Regenerating.	2–3	4–5	4–5	2–3	2–3	

Index